SLEEP TO SAVE YOUR LIFE

Sleep to Save

Your Life

THE COMPLETE GUIDE TO LIVING
LONGER AND HEALTHIER
THROUGH RESTORATIVE SLEEP

Gerard T. Lombardo, M.D.

Collins

An Imprint of HarperCollinsPublishers

FIRST COLLINS PAPERBACK EDITION 2006.

Designed by Fritz Metsch
Illustrations by Dennis M. Willman

The Library of Congress has catalogued the hardcover edition as follows:
Lombardo, Gerard T.
    Sleep to save your life : the complete guide to living longer and healthier through restorative sleep / Gerard T. Lombardo.—1st ed.
        p.   cm.
    Includes bibliographical references and index.

    ISBN-13: 978-0-06-074253-9 (hc)
    ISBN-10: 0-06-074253-4 (hc)
    1. Sleep disorders—Popular works.   2. Sleep—Popular works.   I. Title.
RC547.L65   2005
616.8'498—dc22   2005040391

    ISBN-13: 978-0-06-074254-6 (pbk.)
    ISBN-10: 0-06-074254-2 (pbk.)

---

06   07   08   09   10   ❖/RRD   10   9   8   7   6   5   4   3   2   1

To my wife, Daisy,
and our children Erik, Marc, David, and Angela.

The light of my day and peace of my night.

CONTENTS

Acknowledgments ix

Introduction: Why This Book? 1
1: Sleep to Save Your Life 7
2: Asleep on Your Feet? 18
3: Ready to Sleep 35
4: Good Days, Bad Days 50
5: Snoring—Not a Laughing Matter 61
6: Sleep Apnea—When Breathing Stops 82
7: Snoring and Apnea Treatment 105
8: Narcolepsy—When Sleep "Attacks" 128
9: Restless Legs—Pain in Motion 153
10: Insomnia 165
11: "Around Sleep"—The Mysteries of Parasomnias 193
12: "What's the Matter with Kids Today?" 208
13: Unique Changes—Women and Sleep 224

14: Older, Wiser, and Sleepier 240
15: Low Gear—The Problems of Shift Workers 262

Sleep Diaries 279
References 289
Resources 295
Index 297

ACKNOWLEDGMENTS

Over the years, many of my friends, colleagues, and patients have expressed an interest in having me write an easy-to-read book about sleep disorders. All helped to write this book, and while I cannot acknowledge all of them, I am grateful.

Certain individuals must be mentioned since their input was instrumental in bringing this book to fruition.

To my Celtic and Italian grandparents, a proud thank-you for the legacy of a spiritually sound work ethic, which will, I hope, continue to flow through our future generation as it did through Mom and Dad.

The sleep center at New York Methodist Hospital started 15 years ago and has flourished because of the support and guidance offered by the hospital administration and medical leadership. A special thanks to Trustees' Dr. Peter Mastrorocco, the Reverend Richard Parker, and Mr. Edward Dunn for their friendship, wisdom, and advice shared throughout the years.

As part of the Department of Medicine faculty, I have learned an enormous amount from my fellows and residents. Thank you for caring for our patients and for your contributions to education and research.

Thanks to Dr. Charles Pollack, Dr. Lauren Broch, Dr. Daniel Wagner, and all the members of the New York Cornell Westchester and downtown sleep center for making my training in sleep medicine exceptional in every way, and special thanks to Dr. Arthur Spielman, director of research at our center, who has not only contributed to the field of sleep medicine in general but specifically to the care of patients by his teaching of a small army of new sleep doctoral-level fellows. Thank you for this and for your friendship.

To the NYMH sleep center staff, I believe you are the best in your field, and the patient satisfaction survey completed every morning is proof of that.

To my associate Dr. Thomas Russi and Dr. Andrew Tucker, Associate Director of the Sleep Center, thank you for helping to keep not only the practice together but me together.

Thank you to Toni Sciarra, executive editor at Collins, who shared in the vision and enthusiasm of the project, moved things along when necessary, and offered timely and welcome input.

Thanks to colleagues who, with only a minimum of coaxing, critiqued the manuscript, and to Erik Lombardo, Sam Ehrlich and friends, who not only read the manuscript but afforded me years of clinical observation of the weekend sleeping habits of adolescents.

Thank you, Henry Ehrlich, my writing partner. Henry, I can tell you that I slept better knowing such a talented person and friend of 20 years was up working on the book.

To my ultrafabulous, ever-loving wife and soul mate, Daisy Martinez, who has selflessly supported me in all ways through the years and through the writing of this book. I love you.

SLEEP TO SAVE YOUR LIFE

INTRODUCTION: WHY THIS BOOK?

I wrote this book because the problems associated with sleep disorders are very urgent. As the title implies, this subject is a matter of life and death. You'll learn about some of the really serious consequences that ignoring sleep problems can have for you and for the people around you. Even when the threat to your immediate health seems less than urgent, sleep disorders can be very dangerous to the quality of your life—your work life, your school life, your family life, your sex life, and more. The list could go on and on, but I won't talk about it now. Read the rest of the book.

I also wanted to write a book that would be easily understood. During an initial sleep consultation in January of 2003, a patient complained to me that the local library had one book on sleep disorders that was both too technical and too hard to read. He was surprised by this because he had seen articles in the newspaper about sleep and figured that since it was such a hot topic, there must be some good literature for the average person. Just that morning he had read in *Sports*

Illustrated about professional football players' tendency to experience sleep apnea at five times the levels expected in the population at large. "I guess that three hundred pounds with a twenty-two-inch neck, I must have the same trouble they have, Doctor," he said. Not to mention the restless sleep, dry mouth, and headaches he experienced in the morning. "The snoring reaches dangerous levels when I watch football with my friends," he said. He was joking, but in fact, snoring can be so loud that it becomes painful and damaging to people who have to listen to it, as well as to the snorers themselves.

The shortage of information at the library didn't surprise me. Sleep medicine is a fairly new and rapidly evolving specialty. Dream or REM (rapid eye movement) sleep was described for the first time in the 1950s. Even more recently we have learned that REM sleep is accompanied by an inability to move called **atonia**. Ever wondered why you felt paralyzed during a nightmare? You were!

Treatment for sleep disorders is likewise evolving very rapidly. Psychiatrists, psychologists, or neurologists ran the first sleep centers. Now, in addition to these original specialists, centers are typically staffed by a team that includes pulmonologists—lung specialists—like me, psychologists, otolaryngologists (aka ear, nose, and throat specialists), allergists, nutritionists, bariatric surgeons, orthodontists, cardiologists, pediatricians, and gastroenterologists. Each of these has a role to play in improving patients' sleep.

Burgeoning knowledge of sleep disorders is having a profound, and for me gratifying, effect on the medical community at large. I recently received affirmation of this when I got a referral from a gastroenterologist not affiliated with my hospital. A 50-year-old bus driver had been sent to this doctor for a colonoscopy that is routine for men at that age, and as a bonus to the good news about his disease-free colon, the gastroenterologist diagnosed snoring and obstructive sleep apnea.

No, it's not what you're thinking. He didn't *see* any blockage. The colonoscope thankfully does not reach the tonsils or palate. Rather, the diagnosis came from what the doctor *heard*. He administered a sedative to the patient, who nodded off and immediately started snoring a wet, sloppy snore. "Sawing logs" accompanied by full pauses in his breathing were clear indicators of a sleep disorder called **obstructive sleep apnea (OSA)**. When the patient woke up, the doctor told him he needed to see a sleep specialist right away.

What makes this a significant event is that the physician knew enough about sleep apnea to recognize that this man had a serious problem. The message is getting out.

When I started the sleep center a decade and a half ago at Methodist Hospital in Brooklyn, this wasn't the case. Snoring was seen by most doctors primarily as an annoying quirk whose greatest danger was that it kept spouses from getting a good night's sleep. For the spouses' part, interrupted sleep was seen as an annoyance, something they had to put up with, or, unfortunately for the health of their marriages, as a reason to move to another bedroom. Insomnia for whatever reason was viewed as a temporary condition that could be remedied by relieving underlying anxiety or sleeping late on weekends and cutting down on after-dinner coffee.

However, for pulmonologists, the field in which I received my first board certification, the handwriting has been on the wall for a long time. Indeed, by the time I finished training and joined the Pulmonary Division at Methodist Hospital, sleep training had become a mandatory part of the curriculum in our program and most pulmonary training programs. Sleep medicine is a natural extension of medical practice beyond the field of pulmonology. After all, doctors know firsthand from their training the consequences of not getting enough sleep and should be concerned about it for their patients as well. Sleep medicine is now recognized as a separate and unique multidisciplinary specialty and will soon appear as such in every medical directory and health insurance referral guide, and hospital department directory.

For me there were additional, very personal reasons for my fascination with sleep medicine. As you will read, certain sleep disorders played a part in my life and the lives of other family members. These were, thankfully, the kinds of disorders that were not life-threatening and could be "outgrown." Still, there was something about these conditions that led me to wonder about the lives we lead when we are ostensibly at rest, and that curiosity has become my life's work.

Fifteen years ago there were several well-established sleep centers in Manhattan. Not so for Brooklyn—New York City's most heavily populated borough and, with almost 2.5 million people, in effect the nation's fourth largest city—I was able to persuade the administration of the hospital to open our center. We began with a single bed, which could service only 365 patients a year if we were open every day, which we were not. Those first studies were only occasionally paid for by insurance. Today we have six beds and do some 1,200 sleep studies annually—providing a much-needed service for our community. To meet the growing demand in our area another Brooklyn sleep center has since opened. We have a long way to go to reach and treat all those with sleep disorders and more centers and specialists are needed.

Most sleep studies are reimbursable. Insurance companies, increasingly recognizing the links between sleep disorders and other medical costs, are getting more involved.

The Witness and Diagnosis

Sleep medicine relies heavily on a team approach, and since you may be totally unaware of your condition, a key member of your diagnostic team is the daytime or nighttime witness. Your sleep disorders may affect your spouse or bed partner even more than they affect you, day to night. Not only may your snoring be damaging them physically, but equally important, their observations can help us zero in on a diagnosis. Bed partners can be very accurate in predicting severe apnea even without knowing a thing about the condition.

That's why I ask a new patient to bring a witness—their bed partner—along for the initial consultation. You may wake up repeatedly during the night. You may feel lousy the next day. But it's your bed partner who wakes up and watches you choking or gasping for air. It's your daytime partner who sees the effects your nighttime problems have on you and the people around you. If you sleep alone and suspect you have a sleep disorder, the information contained in this book should help you get a peek at your problem through the nighttime and daytime experiences of others described in case presentations.

As seen in cardiovascular disorders, there are genetic factors that must be considered in helping us optimize your health and that of past, present, and future generations. Sleep problems can be a family affair. For example, Dad may well have sleep apnea, but it might be Mom who has noticed that the children have seasonal allergies that upset their sleeping. Since allergies run in families, this may be a key indicator of an allergic condition in Dad that has gone unnoticed or untreated. Furthermore, such testimony from Mom may indicate that greater attention needs to be paid to sleep as part of the kids' general health care. As you will learn in later chapters, good sleep is crucial not only for immediate health and well-being throughout childhood, but contributes to growth at each developmental stage as well.

Frontiers of Sleep Medicine

We are still at the dawn of sleep medicine, but it is exploding as a field. New technology allows us to look at metabolism at the molecular level, and the conversion of light into electrical impulses by a few cells in your eyes. We know about neurotransmitters and hormones that help flip the on-off switch between waking and sleep.

Some day, we may be able optimize these neurochemical pathways and fix certain sleep disorders the way you can change a fuse after you overload your house electrical system. For now, however, if you are one of the millions of people who suffer from narcolepsy—and go a decade or more without diagnosis—or from insomnia, you have to learn how to efficiently manage wake-time energy and use caution when you operate the washer, dryer, and air-conditioner all at the same time. This book will help.

We are also learning that there are both behavioral and minute chemical links between sleep disorders and such problems as attention-deficit/hyperactivity disorder and psychiatric conditions such as depression. Yet, the medical profession has not yet come to grips with the interrelationships between these conditions and the chemistry involved. While many tantalizing discoveries still lie ahead, we have no choice but to pursue treatment with the chemical, behavioral, and technological tools at hand.

Even the current state of sleep medicine is exciting. I am not alone in believing that sleep medicine is the missing link in treating many of the banes of modern life—hypertension, heart disease, diabetes, and other physical ailments. Why are smoking, substance abuse, overeating, lack of exercise, and disease related to a toxic environment only daytime phenomena? Certainly you bring all of this baggage with you when you get into bed. You are what you eat, sleep, and drink.

A favorite photo of mine is a shot from the 1968 Apollo 8 mission showing earth suspended in our universe, half lit and half in darkness. In a single snapshot we are reminded of the powerful conditions that totally define our human experience—wake and sleep. Arguably sleep can be considered the more important of the two. Sleep well to live well. Sleep to save your life.

I hope that this book will help patients, patients' families, and their family doctors begin to look at the one-third of their lives they spend with their eyes closed as the key to a happier, more productive existence during the two-thirds they spend with their eyes open.

1
_____

SLEEP TO SAVE YOUR LIFE

This test is offered on the New York Methodist Hospital Web site (www.nym.org), to help those seeking information on sleep disorders. (See page 17 for scoring.)

Which statements describe symptoms you have experienced?

1. I do not look forward to sleep because I always have trouble sleeping.
2. Thoughts flood my mind and prevent me from sleeping.
3. I frequently wake up in the middle of the night and can't go back to sleep.
4. I wake up too early in the morning.
5. I worry and have trouble relaxing.
6. I lie awake for at least half an hour before I can fall asleep.
7. I am sad and depressed; I am afraid to fall asleep.

8. Although I can sleep through the night, during the day when I am still awake, I feel muscle tension, crawling sensations, or aching in my legs.
9. Except when I exercise, I feel sleepy during the day.
10. My legs hurt at night and feel better when I move them.
11. I have been told that I kick at night.
12. Sometimes I can't keep my legs still at night. I feel that I have to keep them moving.
13. When I wake up, my muscles are sore and achy.
14. I use antacids (Rolaids, Tums, Alka-Seltzer, etc.) frequently for stomach upset and wake up at night with heartburn.
15. I am hoarse in the morning.
16. I have a chronic cough.
17. I wake up at night wheezing or coughing.
18. I often have sore throats.
19. I'm told that I snore loudly.
20. Although I don't remember it when I wake up, I'm told that while I'm asleep I stop breathing or gasp for breath.
21. I have high blood pressure.
22. My friends or family say they have noticed changes in my personality, along with more daytime sleepiness.
23. I have gained weight.
24. I sweat a great deal during the night.
25. My heart seems to pound or beat irregularly during the night.
26. I get headaches in the morning.
27. I am losing my sex drive.
28. No matter how hard I try to stay awake during the day, I often fall asleep—even if I've had a full night's sleep.
29. When I feel anger, fear, surprise, or other strong emotions, I get a weak feeling in my knees, jaw, or other muscles.
30. Sleepiness is a problem during work or at school.
31. While falling asleep or shortly afterward, I experience vivid, dreamlike scenes.
32. I sometimes fall asleep during physical effort.
33. I feel as if I need to do a full day's work every hour in order to accomplish anything, because I worry about falling asleep.
34. I feel drowsy when driving, even if I've had a full night's sleep.
35. I often feel paralyzed for brief periods while falling asleep or just after waking up.

Some of the questions in this test may surprise you because they may not appear related to sleep disorders. Yet, it is exactly that counterintuitive element that makes sleep such a challenge. Taken one at a time, the symptoms described in this questionnaire may seem like isolated problems that can be dealt with individually—or things that we and the people around us just have to put up with, as we always have.

Taken together, however, they constitute the pieces of a major health puzzle for individuals, for their families, for their coworkers, and for innocent drivers on the highway or others at the mercy of a sleep-deprived person's decisions or actions. Sleep deficiency has been cited in many of the most prominent mishaps of our age, including the Exxon Valdez oil spill, the chemical plant disaster in Bhopal, India, and the destruction of space shuttle *Challenger.* The nuclear power plant disasters at Chernobyl in Ukraine and at Three Mile Island in Pennsylvania, in which millions of lives were jeopardized, took place between one and four o'clock in the morning, when the attention spans of even veteran night shift workers would be suffering most.

The U.S. conflict in Iraq has demonstrated the need for greater focus on sleep management: The *Los Angeles Times* has reported that soldiers occasionally fall asleep behind the wheel of armored vehicles, creating bottlenecked convoys. The U.S. Army has long been concerned with sleeplessness and has tackled the subject head-on with programs such as the one titled "Sustaining Performance during Continuous Operations: The U.S. Army's Sleep Management System" (generated at the Proceedings of the Army Conference in 2000.) Research in this area is covered in Chapter 4, "Good Days, Bad Days."

Every day, similar mishaps occur on the nation's highways and in its factories, often with tragic results, although they usually don't make headlines.

Ultimately, however, a far more insidious public health threat lies in the fact that many of us are dying a slow death because of untreated sleep disorders.

Big Numbers

The numbers of people with sleep problems of all kinds are alarming and very costly for society at large.

One comprehensive survey, conducted in 1997 by Louis Harris and Associates, Inc., on behalf of the National Sleep Foundation (NSF), estimated that sleep problems from a variety of sources afflict nearly half of employed adults and that two-thirds of these, or 36 million, have trouble making it through the day as a result.

Sixty-three percent reported having difficulty handling stress. Sixty percent claimed to have difficulty concentrating. Fifty-seven percent had trouble listening to what others were saying, and many had difficulty solving problems, making decisions, and relating to coworkers. The study estimates the cost of sleep loss on employers at some $18 billion.

Asked how much sleeplessness affects different aspects of their lives, 19 percent said it affects their overall health "very much," 46 percent said "somewhat," while 21 percent said it affects their ability to pursue personal interests very much and 43 percent said it affects their personal interests somewhat.

Sixty percent said sleeplessness affects their work life— 14 percent very much and 46 percent somewhat. Fifty-eight percent claimed sleeplessness affects their personal relationships—18 percent very much and 40 percent somewhat. And 51 percent blamed it for compromising their ability to pursue career goals—17 percent very much and 34 percent somewhat. That's a whole lot of life that is being damaged.

A 1999 study published in the journal *Sleep* concluded that the mean annual medical tab for patients with undiagnosed sleep apnea was $2,720, compared with $1,384 for those without sleep apnea— more than double the cost. The estimated additional medical costs were $3.4 billion.

Another study of 97 newly diagnosed sleep apnea patients and an equal number of subjects who don't have sleep apnea showed that those with apnea spent 251 nights in the hospital over a two-year period before diagnosis, compared with 90 nights for the control group. And that's just for a two-year period. Presumably they were paying higher costs much earlier. Given the prevalence of sleep apnea, how much money and how many lives could be saved if early screening was done for apnea on the same scale as for colon cancer or breast cancer? Add to that lost productivity at work for patients and their spouses, domestic stress, and diminished quality of life and, to quote the late Senator Everett Dirksen, "pretty soon you're talking about real money."

The extent of treatment is still minor.

Even with our capacity at New York Methodist of 1,200 sleep studies per year, we're barely scratching the surface. If, as we now estimate, 4 percent of the population suffers from sleep apnea—a level comparable with asthma—in Brooklyn alone we're talking about nearly 100,000 cases, enough to keep local sleep specialists busy for 100 years. It's exhausting just to think about it. Nationwide, we're talking about 12 to 18 million people affected directly, compounded by serious secondary effects on the people they sleep with, work with, and drive with.

Sleep apnea is now recognized as a significant cofactor—an accompanying condition or contributing cause—for a growing number of diseases: asthma, coronary artery disease, congestive heart failure, depression, diabetes, hypertension—a regular murderers' row. That means that sleep apnea belongs on a list that includes smoking, heavy drinking, obesity, and lack of exercise as a serious danger to long-term health.

Day Doctors and Night Doctors

General medical practice has been a little slow to catch up on the explosive growth of new information in the field of sleep medicine. Sleep is still frequently overlooked as a factor in the treatment of many serious conditions. Take high blood pressure. When a patient with high blood pressure goes to the doctor for a *daytime* appointment, the condition may well be under control because he took medication first thing in the morning. There is no need to consider what goes on at night—or is there?

If he has untreated sleep apnea, his blood pressure and heart rate may shoot up hundreds of times a night. The effects on the heart, the lungs, the vascular system, and the nervous system are serious, and expensive to treat.

That's where a sleep medicine evaluation can help. The need for such an evaluation may be obvious to you or your doctor if the symptoms are severe enough. For more subtle conditions doctors are relying on short questionnaires designed to screen for medical and sleep disorders. These may be filled out in the waiting room while you wait for your visit. One example of such a screening tool is the Epworth Sleepiness Scale presented at the beginning of Chapter 4.

Once a sleep disorder is suspected, it is our job to evaluate the history, confirm the diagnosis or order appropriate tests, and recommend treatment. By making sleep safe and efficient, we can help your doctor's treatment become more effective, saving you a lot of misery, and your insurance company a lot of money.

Sleep medicine is an essential component of 24-hour medicine.

$47 Billion and Counting!

What is the overall cost of sleep apnea to the nation?

- Consider that individuals with moderate to severe sleep apnea are 4.5 times as likely to have coronary heart disease, myocardial infarction, and angina as are those without sleep apnea.
- Twenty-three percent of new cases of these diseases—over 41,000 per year—are associated with sleep apnea, a rate that could be drastically reduced if apnea was more aggressively treated. As it is, just 1 percent of all obstructive sleep apnea patients are receiving treatment. How does this affect the nation's health bill?
- If someone with chest pain receives a successful angioplasty, tests and treatment could cost about $30,000. If the angioplasty is unsuccessful and the patient has a heart attack, the costs will rise as high as $100,000 or more.
- Diagnosis and treatment of obstructive sleep apnea costs between $1,000 and $3,000.
- A study of physician costs after sleep-apnea treatment found that they were 33 percent lower, and there were 50 percent fewer hospitalizations among patients who stuck to their prescribed treatment.

Depending on the medical results, identifying and treating those thousands of new patients could save more than $47 billion annually. And that's just sleep apnea!

24/7

Then there are the problems created by our 24/7-business environment. An estimated 20 to 25 percent of our labor force is now doing some sort of shift work, and the number is growing by 3 percent per year. What this means is that one out of every four workers is fighting an inborn physical schedule, which evolved over millions of years, of working when it's light and sleeping when it's dark. Their individual problems are compounded by their need to interact with family members who keep to traditional schedules. Sleep time loses out.

Sleep and Weight

Many of us are concerned about our weight, and we are bombarded with alarming statistics about the rising incidence of obesity, as well as methods to lose weight that seem to be too good to be true, which they probably are.

The evidence is that this trend has a strong link to sleep deprivation. A study of 18,000 subjects led by Dr. Steven Heymsfield of Columbia University and St. Luke's–Roosevelt Hospital in New York and James Gangwisch, a Columbia epidemiologist, found that those who got less than seven to nine hours of sleep were substantially more likely to be obese than those who got the recommended amount. The risks multiply in nice, neat numbers as people get less sleep than they should. Those who got six hours had a 23 percent greater chance of being obese, while those who averaged five hours of sleep had 50 percent greater risk. Those who got four hours of sleep a night were 73 percent more likely to be obese!

There's a chicken and egg problem here. Are people obese because they don't sleep or are people not sleeping because they are obese? As you will read in Chapters 5 and 6, there's a definite linkage between being overweight and sleep disordered breathing, particularly sleep apnea. However, as Dr. Heymsfield said, "There's growing scientific evidence that there's a link between sleep and the various neural pathways that regulate food intake." The sleep-deprived have lower levels of a blood protein called leptin, which helps the body determine when it has eaten enough. At the same time, levels of ghrelin, which makes people want to eat, rise.

Some of the links between being overweight and sleeplessness are indirect. For example, overweight patients will complain about pain in their knees and ankles. Any such persistent pain is going to cause trouble at night, and compromise the quality of your sleep.

Whatever the relationship between sleep deprivation and weight gain, treatment of one will be more effective if the other is treated at the same time.

Sleep to Save the Lives of Other People

Then there are the effects of sleepiness on the nation's highways. More than half of American drivers say that they have driven while drowsy during the past year, and 19 percent have actually fallen asleep at the wheel.

Legislators have taken note and are responding with new laws. This movement came in response to the death in 1997 of a 20-year-old college student, Maggie McDonnell, in New Jersey. A car crossed three lanes of highway traffic and hit Maggie's car head-on. The driver confessed that he had been awake for 30 hours and using drugs before the accident. At the first trial, the jury deadlocked 9 to 3 for conviction. In the second, the defense argued that New Jersey had no law against falling asleep at the wheel, and therefore the driver did nothing wrong. He received a suspended jail sentence and a $200 fine.

On June 23, 2003, the New Jersey State Senate passed a bill known as "Maggie's Law," which establishes fatigued driving as recklessness under the existing vehicular homicide statute, the first such law in the nation. It defines "fatigue" as being without sleep for more than 24 consecutive hours.

Also in 2003, the U.S. House of Representatives introduced a law at the federal level, citing these estimates (described in the bill as conservative) for the year 1995:

- 100,000 police-reported motor vehicle crashes caused by the drowsiness or fatigue of the operator
- 1,550 deaths and 71,000 injuries resulting directly from a driver falling asleep at the wheel of a motor vehicle
- $12 billion, the cost of these crashes in diminished productivity and property loss

BREAKER, BREAKER. TAKE A SLEEP BREAK!

Sleepy truckers have been a safety concern since the hours-of-service (HOS) regulations were first implemented in 1939. Thankfully, the rules were revised in April 2003 by the Federal Motor Carrier Safety Administration (FMCSA) in cooperation with trucking locals and the U.S. secretary of transportation. The update was long overdue considering the startling statistics on truck-related motor vehicle accidents.

Jim Hall, then chairman of the National Transportation Safety Board (NTSB), told the Parents Against Tired Truckers:

- Forty-two thousand people die and another 3.5 million people are injured in traffic crashes on American roads every year.
- Annual monetary costs to society exceed $150 billion.
- Trucks are overrepresented in these numbers. In 1997, large

trucks accounted for about 3 percent of all registered vehicles and 8 percent of total vehicle miles traveled.

- Thirteen percent of all traffic fatalities that year occurred in crashes involving large trucks.
- Of the 5,355 people killed in crashes involving large trucks in 1997, 78 percent were occupants of another vehicle.
- Of the 133,000 people injured in these crashes, 75 percent were in another vehicle.

The NTSB has instituted new standards of enforcement for the nation's long-distance truckers. For years, the recommended standard has been eight hours of uninterrupted sleep during a ten-hour break following a ten-hour drive. Now with the new rulings in force, all parties will be liable. In addition, there is a proposal for mandatory electronic devices to log the vehicle's hours on the road. An added and not often mentioned potential benefit will be improved overall health and safety of our "big buddies."

Sleep to Save Your Quality of Life

In addition to the major life-and-death elements of sleep disorders, there are also sleep problems such as narcolepsy and restless legs syndrome that afflict huge numbers of Americans and that can make your life miserable. Indeed in the case of narcolepsy, which, briefly, is an uncontrollable urge to sleep during the waking day, the effects on your quality of life are as negative as those of Hodgkin's disease, multiple sclerosis, and other crippling and life-threatening illnesses. While symptoms of narcolepsy can strike at any age, the peak years of onset are between 15 and 30, which means that it exerts a huge drag on some of the most formative and productive years of life.

Despite the fact that both restless legs and narcolepsy afflict significant percentages of Americans, they are generally undiagnosed for a decade or more on average, causing substantial needless physical and psychological suffering. Furthermore, those who are diagnosed represent a very small fraction of those who actually have these conditions. The rest go untreated, self-treated, or wrongly treated. While there are no definitive treatments for these conditions, they can be managed in ways that will minimize their potential for chronic misery.

My great hope is that reading the sections on these conditions in this book will spark recognition among the silent sufferers, who can then seek state-of-the-art treatment. I don't pretend that this book is the *last* word on these conditions. Sleep medicine is a work in progress. But I hope that it is an effective *first* word for many people who know that something is wrong and don't know what it is. I hope that they will recognize their symptoms and seek treatment. They are not alone, but they may think they are. Tens of millions of Americans suffer from diagnosable sleep conditions but somehow think they are unique, and that the only thing to be done is to drink more coffee to stay awake, fake it at work and school, drink alcohol at night to go to sleep, and so on. Sleep disorders are not a hopeless fact of modern life. They are medical conditions that can be treated, even if they cannot always be "cured."

Sleep Deprivation—the Next Generation

We are also raising a generation of sleep-deprived children. In addition to the demands of school, Internet chat lines, junk food snacking, lack of physical activity, and sleep bingeing on weekends, our teenagers are stunting their physical and mental growth by neglecting their sleep hygiene and falling asleep in class. And those are just the "normal" ones. Then there are those with undiagnosed disorders such as narcolepsy and restless legs, which exact a price in morale, social development, and many other measures of mental health.

As you will read, more attention is being paid to the way hospital nurseries are run precisely because of the susceptibility of infant brains to organic disruption in those first critical hours after a baby goes from floating in the peace and security of the womb to the world of light, noise, gravity, and people.

When you examine some of these factors in childhood, you can begin to see where behavior patterns and habits formed early in life can lead to sleep disorders later in life, both organic disease and problems psychological in nature. Sorting them out and treating them is thus a complicated process. Specific conditions now number over 70, including insomnia, narcolepsy, neurological diseases, movement disorders of the limbs, and parasomnias, including sleepwalking and sleep talking. Add to that common and epidemic conditions known to be associated with disordered breathing at night, like childhood obesity, and the numbers of children affected keep going up.

That is why our 14-doctor multidisciplinary team at the sleep center includes practitioners in a wide range of specialties along with six polysomnography technicians and four to five sleep medicine doctoral candidates.

During a night's stay at our hotel-style rooms, complete with generous-sized beds and cable TV to make the stay as homelike as possible, our technicians monitor 15 body activities, including brain waves, oxygen levels, carbon dioxide levels, airflow, rapid eye movement (REM), chest and abdomen movement, muscle activity in the chin and legs, heart rate, and of course snoring.

But you don't need all these people to know if you have a problem or to begin to treat it. I hope you took the test at the beginning of this chapter. Below are the "answers." After you evaluate yourself, you can begin to take commonsense measures to start back on the road to rest, and to health.

How Did You Do?

Questions 1–7 describe the symptoms experienced by people who have insomnia, the persistent inability to fall asleep or stay asleep.

Questions 8–13 describe the symptoms experienced by people who have nocturnal limb movement disorder, or restless legs syndrome, disorders characterized by abnormal movements, aching, or crawling sensations in the legs or sometimes arms.

Questions 14–18 describe the symptoms experienced by people with gastroesophageal reflux, a disorder that results from stomach acid backing up into the throat during the night.

Questions 19–27 describe the symptoms experienced by people who have sleep apnea, a potentially life-threatening disorder that causes one to stop breathing repeatedly (possibly hundreds of times) during sleep.

Questions 28–35 describe the symptoms experienced by people with narcolepsy, a complex disorder with uncontrollable sleep attacks during the day as one of its symptoms.

If the answer to any or many of these questions is yes, you or your loved one may be on their way to a lifetime of medical misery unless you do something about it.

2

ASLEEP ON YOUR FEET?

Sleep that knits up the ravelled sleave of care,
The death of each day's life, sore labour's bath,
Balm of hurt minds, great nature's second course,
Chief nourisher in life's feast.

—William Shakespeare, *Macbeth*

Despite the fact that sleep has always been a central concern of mankind, most of what we know about sleep we have learned in the last 50 years or so.

Why Do We Sleep?

For thousands of years, sleep was thought of as a comalike opposite of wakefulness—"The death of each day's life." However, while people like Shakespeare may have understood intuitively that a good night's sleep was good for us—"Chief nourisher in life's feast"—how sleep worked was beyond us until the mid–20th century.

Certainly there was one sleep phenomenon that was recognized early in civilization—dreaming. Remember that, according to the Bible, when Joseph was sold into bondage in Egypt, he gained favor with the pharaoh because he could interpret his dreams. Dr. Sigmund Freud saw dreams as a window into unresolved psychological conflict and therefore as a component of mental health, but he couldn't study their connection to pathways in the brain because there was no way at that time to chart the brain's behavior during sleep.

That began to change in the early 1950s when the electroencephalogram (EEG) technology was applied to sleep.

Now, thanks to our knowledge of brain waves, we know that most dreaming takes place during a stage of sleep called **rapid eye movement,** or **REM, sleep.** We also know that REM is not only critical for psychological reasons but we strongly suspect that it plays a central role in maintaining a healthy body. Consider that rats, which have a normal life span of two to three years, survive only about five weeks on average when they don't get any REM sleep. When deprived of all sleep stages, they live only about three weeks. They also suffer from an inability to regulate body temperatures, and develop sores on their tails and paws, possibly because sleeplessness damages their immune systems.

Returning to the human animal, it is clear that rather than representing a mere absence of consciousness, the sleeping body is a cauldron of activity necessary for functioning in the "real" waking world. REM sleep is a riot of electrical impulses so intense that if it happened when you were awake, you wouldn't be able to function. When do stock exchanges, banks, and other complex computer systems operators upgrade and test their equipment? At the height of their working day? No. They wait until their customers have gone home for the night. Your brain functions in much the same way.

Profile of a Normal Night's Sleep

SLEEP STAGES OF ADULTS

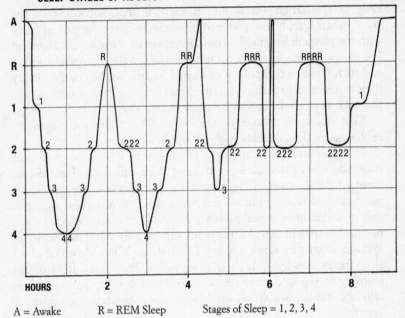

A = Awake   R = REM Sleep   Stages of Sleep = 1, 2, 3, 4

LIGHT NON-REM SLEEP

Stage 1. We drift into sleep and are easily reawakened. During this stage we may experience a **hypnic jerk**—the kind of sudden "startle" reflex similar to what we experience when we start to fall. As we sink deeper into sleep, our eyes move very slowly and our muscle activity slows.

Stage 2. Our eye movements stop and brain waves slow down, with occasional bursts of rapid waves.

People awakened after more than a few minutes of sleep are usually unable to recall the last few minutes before they nodded off. This declining ability to remember as our sleep deepens is called **sleep-related amnesia.** That is why phone calls or conversations that we had late at night are forgotten in the morning, and why when we turn off our alarm clocks and go back to sleep, we can't remember that we did so.

Stage 3. Brain waves continue to slow and deep sleep waves, or **delta waves,** begin to appear, interspersed with smaller, faster waves.

Stage 4. The brain switches to almost total delta, deep wave, sleep. It is very difficult to wake someone during stages 3 and 4. Children have a higher proportion of stage-3 and -4 sleep, when compared with adults.

SLEEP STAGES OF CHILDREN

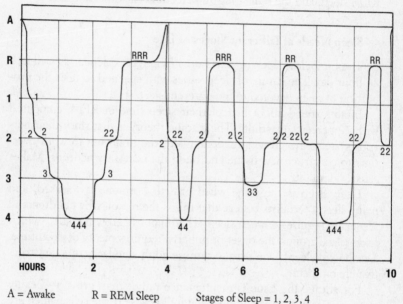

A = Awake   R = REM Sleep   Stages of Sleep = 1, 2, 3, 4

Eye movement and muscle activity are reduced during deep sleep. When awakened, people do not adjust immediately and often feel groggy and disoriented. During deep sleep, children sometimes wet their beds, experience night terrors, or sleepwalk.

REM SLEEP

Our breathing speeds up or becomes irregular and shallow. Our eyes jerk rapidly in various directions—hence the name rapid eye movement. Our arm and leg muscles become temporarily paralyzed, which keeps us from acting out our dreams; the heart rate increases; blood pressure rises; and both men and women experience changes in erectile tissue.

A complete sleep cycle averages 90 to 110 minutes. The first burst of REM sleep usually happens about 70 to 90 minutes after we fall asleep. The first sleep cycles each night have short REM periods and long periods of deep sleep. As the night goes on, REM sleep periods lengthen and deep sleep shortens. By morning, people spend nearly all their sleep time in stages 1, 2, and REM. Overall, adults spend almost 50 percent of their total sleep time in stage 2 sleep, about 20 percent in REM sleep, and the remaining 30 percent in the other stages.

Sleep Needs at Different Stages of Life

The biological clock operates on a long-term calendar as well as a 24-hour day. The nature of sleep varies with age, and so does the proportion of sleep devoted to the different sleep stages.

Infants spend about half of their sleep time in REM, compared with 20 percent for adults. The leading theory is that since their nervous systems are growing exponentially, the brain has to work overtime to construct new tissue and build the necessary neurons. Makes sense, doesn't it?

Deep sleep is the stage when growth hormone is released, and many sleep specialists believe that this is the reason why children and teenagers require so much sleep. That famous "growth spurt," which takes place around the onset of puberty, requires plenty of downtime. Let the kid sleep! Don't try to impose adult standards of a constructive life on them.

For adults, the issue is maintenance rather than growth—beauty sleep, in effect. Why do adults need it? Because tissue cells, which are worn out during the normal wear and tear of living, need sleep to repair themselves. People who live too hard show it in their faces—bags under the eyes, wrinkles, lack of skin tone. If all that is happening on the surface, think about the parts of the body you can't see. That's where all those linkages between sleep and conditions like heart disease, diabetes, and stroke come into play. When you don't get enough good-quality sleep, your vital organs and other tissues are not getting the healthy doses of scheduled repair and vital hormones they need to restore their capacity to do their work.

Deep sleep also has a profound effect on your waking mental state. Parts of the brain that control emotions, decision-making processes, and social interactions appear to be quiet during deep sleep, suggesting that they need time off to recover from the stresses and strains of waking life.

Memories

Don't know much about history? Maybe you would if you had made a point of getting a good night's sleep after studying when you were in school.

Another study of rats showed that certain nerve-signaling patterns recorded during the day were repeated during deep sleep. Does your brain need to replay events so that you will remember them? I know from my own experience as a student that what I learned pulling all-nighters to cram for exams was not retained as well as what I studied in a more rested state.

Think about that when you pay your kid's college tuition!

Keys to Your Sleeping Problems
WHAT'S WRONG WITH YOUR LIFE?

When new patients come to see me to get help with a sleep disorder, the first thing I ask them is, more or less, "What's wrong with your life?" I ask them to talk about their day as a 24-hour cycle. For many of them it's the first time a health care question has been framed in terms of a *full* day.

I need to get an idea of what *they* think the sleep problem is. If they have trouble falling asleep or staying asleep and the lack of sleep is dominating their thinking, that by definition is insomnia, which is discussed in detail in Chapter 10. Often they suspect something is wrong because they are tired or lack energy during the day. If there is no witness to tell them about their sleep behavior, I make it a point to ask specific questions that can elicit evidence of a problem.

Most of us think that what goes on in the daytime is more important than what goes on at night. We put up with sleep problems as long as we can because the day defines who we are. Practically no one goes to see a sleep doctor until something happens during the day that bothers them so much they can't put it off any longer. As the problem starts to affect their waking life regularly, they begin to worry; when it gets really bad, they go to the doctor. They are losing the ability to be what they want to be.

Okay. I know I have described *four* stages of sleep above, but for purposes of answering the big question, *what's wrong with your life?*, I'm going divide your 24-hour day into *three* parts: the time you are awake, REM sleep, and non-REM sleep. This way it is easier to explain certain things.

When something goes wrong in one of these three areas, it shows up somewhere else, like a bubble in the carpet. You step on the bubble and it moves. You are only displacing it. What you really have to do is go to the edge of the carpet and pull on it.

Your daytime problems are like the moving bubble. They are waking symptoms of problems you have when you sleep. Likewise, your nighttime problems may result from problems you have during the day. They may be physical, psychological, or behavioral in origin.

If you find yourself yawning and dozing off during the day, very likely there's something wrong at night, but you may not know anything about it. If you can't sleep at night, you may well be under too much stress during the day, not getting enough exercise, not eating right, or your physical health may be suffering. Whatever the problem, by the time you get to a sleep specialist, your body is signaling, "Houston, we have a problem."

There are as many answers to the question, *what's wrong with your life?*, of course, as the number of people who consult me.

For example, there was the bus driver who said, "I'm going to lose my job."

Or the schoolteacher who said, "I can't get through a day in the classroom without dozing off."

Or the banker who claimed, "There's nothing wrong with me, but my wife keeps complaining that I snore."

Or the young wife who came in with her husband who had fresh bruises and scratches on his chest and hands and said, "I keep doing this to him while I'm asleep. I have to stop."

Or the retired executive secretary who said simply, "I can't sleep!"

Or the middle-aged man on disability who said, "Nothing is wrong with my sleep, but my doctor told me to come here."

Once we answer the question of what's wrong, that's just the tip of the iceberg. The challenge to patient and doctor is to find out what's under the surface of a patient's symptoms and treat it before disaster strikes. This is no exaggeration. Life and death and quality of life hang in the balance.

When that bus driver said to me, "I'm going to lose my job," he was distilling a complicated set of circumstances to the most basic level. He works in a very stressful job, requiring constant use of both body and mind. He may have to drive for hours every day in congested New York City streets. He has to contend with the bad habits of other drivers, potholes, and irritable passengers and still safely drive the bus. He may be sitting down, but every muscle is in constant use. This is a man who earns a good night's sleep. He needs to recover from the stresses of the day. What happens when he cannot get his rest? His back hurts. His head aches. He yawns while trying to steer a 50-foot bus in and out of traffic.

His symptoms distract him from the task at hand, which is to deliver working people to their jobs, shoppers to stores, and young people to and from school. Lives are in jeopardy—not only his own but those of his passengers, other drivers, and pedestrians. His employer's answer, given the fact that he has been dozing at his job, was to suggest that he find another line of work. He came to me in the hope of avoiding that eventuality. Not only is he good at his job, but his salary and excellent benefits are critical to his family's standard of living.

The problem for me as his physician was to figure out whether his job was taking a toll on his sleep, or whether his sleep problems were taking a toll on his job.

What about the schoolteacher? She, in fact, knew what was wrong with her life. She had been diagnosed with narcolepsy, meaning that she is prone to excessive or uncontrollable sleepiness, which hits her during the middle of the day. This is a bad condition for someone who has to spend seven hours in front of a class of 35 kids, which every parent knows is too many even if you don't have narcolepsy. She had tried very hard to have her condition treated and nothing seemed to work. She came to me because she had heard about a certain new drug for treating her symptoms. I explained the benefits and risks associated with the medication, including potential side effects.

She didn't hesitate. She was willing to take the risk because she wanted to continue teaching. All our children should have such dedicated teachers.

The retired executive secretary has a very different problem. After many years of working, retirement deprived her life of a purpose, and with that void came insomnia. This is a phenomenon that is going to be repeated over and over again as baby boomers retire. The National Sleep Foundation estimates that 30 percent of the 70 million members of the baby-boomer generation will experience this kind of insomnia.

As for the young married woman and her afflicted husband, they are both victims of her **parasomnia,** involuntary activity that takes place during deep sleep. While many people have parasomnia conditions such as sleepwalking, which affects many children, in certain cases the predisposition can combine with stress and anxiety to produce dangerous behavior.

HOW FAR CAN WE PUSH OURSELVES?

Military organizations put a lot of money into extending the waking day. The logic is clear. To paraphrase Rudyard Kipling, if you can stay awake and keep fighting while your enemy falls asleep, you win.

The United States Defense Advanced Research Projects Agency (DARPA) is hoping to find ways for soldiers to stay awake for up to a week.

Current drugs just won't do for DARPA, so the organization is looking to some highly unconventional sources for possible solutions, from magnetic resonance imagery (MRI) studies to map and possibly treat sleepy sections of the brain, to studies of birds to see how they manage to keep flying for days at a time during migration, to scans of dolphins' brains to see how they manage to sleep with part of their brains while continuing to perform tasks like rising to the surface to breathe.

Yaakov Stern and Sarah Lisanby, researchers at Columbia University with funding from DARPA, are using MRI to identify parts of the brain that perform critical mental tasks. Eventually they will use transcranial magnetic stimulation (TMS) on sleep-deprived soldiers to trigger neurons in those parts of the brain to see if they can improve performance. TMS has been effective in some studies in treating severe depression.

However, there are surely limits to humans' ability to manipulate their sleep needs. Charles Heyman, an ex–army major who now works as a military consultant, says, "What you see is people's reactions becoming impaired, their ability to make decisions is affected, and before long they are absolutely no use to you." Tests conducted at the Walter Reed Army Institute of Research in Silver Spring, Maryland, show that physical and thinking ability diminishes an average of 25 percent for every 24 hours without sleep.

(Sources: Amanda Onion,abcnews.go.com/Technology/story?id=97805&page=1; Ian Sample, *The Guardian,* July 29, 2004)

Most people who come to see me know there's something wrong with them, but sometimes those who believe they don't have a problem really do have one. Take the case of the banker who said, "There's nothing wrong with me, but my wife keeps complaining that I snore." He went on to say, "I'm fully alert at work. I travel a lot and do multimillion-dollar deals without ever getting jet lag. I work long hours. When my head hits the pillow, I'm gone until morning."

I asked him, "You feel fine, but how does your wife feel?"

"Well," he said, "she says that my snoring keeps waking her up and sometimes she sleeps on the couch."

"Let's take this one thing at a time," I told him. "First of all, even if snoring didn't indicate physical problems for you, isn't marriage hard enough without making your wife miserable?"

"I hadn't thought of that," he said. Then he added, "When she can't sleep, she's impossible."

"Second, your snoring is bad for her health," I said. "It is interrupting her sleep, which keeps her from getting the sleep *she* needs and it may even affect her hearing.

"And third," I added, "snoring can be a sign that something is really wrong with you. Just because you feel fine now doesn't mean you won't have big problems later in life. You can live with a bad heart for years, too, and never know anything's wrong until you keel over."

With these three arguments on the table, he consented to have a sleep study. The study showed that he had sleep apnea, which, as you will read in Chapter 6, can be a destructive chronic condition. I recommended that he use a device called a CPAP (continues positive air pressure) machine to help him breathe at night.

He was stubborn. "I'll have to think it over."

"Sleep on it," I told him. Pun intended.

He didn't surrender without a fight. He called up a few days later and told me triumphantly, "I found a study published online that shows you don't have to treat sleep apnea if you function normally during the day."

"When was the article published?" I asked him.

"Nineteen ninety-one," he replied.

"Tell me," I said. "What kind of computer do you use?" He proudly named a high-end PC with the latest software. I asked, "You wouldn't use a computer manual written in 1991, would you? Well, the science of sleep medicine is growing just as fast as computer technology. That study is way out-of-date."

SUNRISE, SUNSET, AND YOU

To appreciate all the things that can go wrong with your sleeping, it helps to appreciate the multidimensional complexity of your sleep mechanism.

Your body is a remarkable instrument in many ways, not least of which is the schedule it runs on. The term "biological clock" is often used when referring to a woman's childbearing years. In fact, we all—men, women, and children—have a biological clock, which goes by a name that is a lot bigger than it is—**suprachiasmatic nucleus,** or **SCN** for short. The SCN is located in a part of the brain called the **hypothalamus,** just above the point where the optic nerves cross.

Light on the photoreceptors in the retina at the back of your eye is converted into electrical and chemical signals that travel along the optic nerve to the SCN.

Light inhibits the secretion of the hormone melatonin by the pineal gland, which normally peaks between the hours of one to five in the morning, when the night is darkest. By this and other means, your body is conditioned to operate almost exactly on the same schedule as the earth's daily rotation—actually about 25 hours every day instead of 24. Thus, from the word *circadian*—"around a day"—we call this cycle **circadian rhythm.**

Our ancestors' discovery of fire may have been the beginning of the end of a "normal" night's sleep for mankind. The grown-ups could stay up late and sit around the campfire, or take turns watching for wolves.

Regardless, your body still needs to rest on the same caveman schedule. Ever wonder why many countries have a rest period in the middle of the afternoon, best known as a siesta? Maybe you, too, have a groggy spell at 3 P.M. or so. It's part of your circadian rhythm. Some shift workers—those whose schedules are continually disrupted—are throwing sand in the gears of their circadian rhythms.

The 24–25-hour sleep-waking day is just one element in an integrated biological system of timing and balance that can compare with, say, the operation of the world's air traffic control system, or the world financial system, or the North American power grid, only it doesn't require the thousands of people those systems do. However, just as the computers that operate those systems require conscious monitoring and maintenance, so your sleeping mechanism requires a certain amount of human oversight.

DAYLIGHT SAVINGS TIME

"Spring forward . . . fall back."

That little mnemonic device is how many of us remember to set our clocks twice a year when we go on or off daylight saving time. But our bodies are not so quick to adjust and the results can be dangerous.

One survey has shown that traffic accidents surge by 7 percent following the springtime change, when we lose an hour of sleep, and that this effect lasts about a week. While the process reverses itself when we gain an hour in the fall, this is small comfort to those who are injured in the spring.

As much as anything, this statistic should convince any skeptic of the delicacy of their biological clock.

SELF-REGULATION

The need for sleep is remarkably consistent from day to day. If you stay up too late one night and wake up at your usual time in the morning, you have acquired a **sleep deficit**. You feel sleepy the next day and you require more sleep to make up for it. This built-in balancing act is called **sleep homeostasis.** The process is most apparent in many homes because of the behavior of teenage children. They stay up late at night all week running around, talking to their friends on the Internet, or watching TV—after finishing their homework, of course—and then sleep soundly into the early afternoon on weekends. I was most acutely aware of this when my eldest son came home from college. Anyone can acquire a sleep deficit. One late night does not a sleep disorder make. But if you burn the midnight oil night after night, or if something happens to you while you are sleeping that disrupts the rest and restorative qualities of sleep, you will suffer from one or more significant health problems.

SLEEP DEPRIVATION AND YOUR BRAIN

With the help of **positron-emission tomography,** popularly known as **PET scan,** doctors can now see how hard parts of our brains are working. A small measure of a radioactive substance called **radionuclide** is combined with a sugar and injected into the patient. The radioactive material emits particles called **positrons,** and the PET scanner rotates around the patient's head to detect emissions of these particles. Thus, we can see evidence of tumor growth, because tumor tissue metabolizes glucose at different rates than healthy brain tissue. We can also see the brain change as it hatches ideas, although we cannot tell what the ideas are about. PET scans tell a very bleak story about the effects of sleep deprivation on the brain. Studies show that after staying awake for only 24 hours, the metabolic activity of the brain diminishes up to 6 percent for the whole brain and up to 11 percent for specific areas of brain function. Can you do without 6 percent or more of your brain function?

Glucose-PET studies show that sleep deprivation for 24 hours reduces metabolism in the areas that are most important for judgment, impulse control, attention, and visual association.

How does this affect your life? The first casualties are tasks that require both speed and accuracy. People who need eight hours of sleep per night who are allowed to sleep for only seven hours a night over the space of a week are slower at tasks that demand both simple reaction time and mathematical-problem-solving abilities, although they are still accurate. On sleep of just five hours a night for a week, their accuracy starts to go, too.

More complex tasks suffer greatly when the sleep deprivation continues for more than a week. In driving simulations, for example, the number of accidents rises progressively as sleep is decreased to seven, five, and three hours. In these tests, three hours of total sleep resulted in the loss of the ability to process peripheral vision and the incidence of recklessness rises as people lose their ability to appreciate the possible consequences of their actions.

REM AND NON-REM—SPECIAL STATES WITH SPECIAL FUNCTIONS

Have you ever watched a dog or a cat sleep? Every so often they start to twitch. Their eyes under the closed eyelids begin to move rapidly in all directions. You can easily imagine that your dog is dreaming about chasing a squirrel, or the cat is dreaming about stalking a bird.

The eye movements are caused by alternating cycles of REM sleep, the same as with people.

REM and non-REM sleep have some things in common with one another. In both you are relatively still and unaware of what is going on around you. However, the differences between them are dramatic.

During REM sleep, much of your brain is more active than it is when you are awake. The best evidence of the extent of REM brain activity is the vividness of your dreams, which can include sight, sound, smell—all the senses at once. *Star Wars* can't match them for special effects, and your freewheeling dreaming imagination is a match for any screenwriter. Our dreams can be comedy, tragedy, or horror, although most of us can't convert them into movies. Your dreams can incorporate material not only from your everyday concerns but also—as Dr. Freud believed—from your suppressed wake-time experiences.

The innate genius of REM sleep is particularly evident in those horror movies that we call nightmares. Have you ever fallen off a cliff in a dream, or been chased by a monster? Were you ever so scared that you struggled to wake yourself up only to find that you couldn't move? That's because you couldn't. You were paralyzed.

And it's a good thing, too. You wouldn't want your mechanic to adjust the timing on your car when it's in gear. The car would go right through the wall and probably take the mechanic with it. If your voluntary muscles weren't paralyzed during REM sleep, you would probably run through the wall and take your bed partner with you.

Not all your muscles are immobilized, of course. Those that assist the actions of your heart and lungs, for example, must continue to function, although, as I will describe later in the chapter on sleep apnea, your body is in real danger if they are interrupted.

WHEN IS A "SLEEP PROBLEM" NOT A PROBLEM?

A weird schedule doesn't mean you have a sleeping problem, per se. We can get a full night's (or day's) rest even with unconventional hours, as long as the hours are uninterrupted and the different cycles have a chance to play themselves out.

Take the case of a man I'll call Bill. He had been a skilled machinist, but years ago he broke his ankle in a job accident, which greatly restricted his mobility. Fortunately, he had extensive permanent disability coverage. Unlike many of us, he also had avid interests, which he could pursue when it became clear after a series of surgeries that he would never be able to ply his trade again.

A new GP referred him to me. This was a positive sign—the doctor was aware that there is a field called sleep medicine.

Bill claimed that there was nothing wrong with his life. However, since he slept alone, I was convinced that he was one of the many patients who were unaware of their sleep disorder. Funny thing, though.

Bill was right. His doctor was worried because Bill couldn't get to sleep until 3 A.M. every night. To the doctor, that was a problem.

However, it was the same time every night, and it followed several hours of quiet, totally absorbed work on his hobby, coin collecting. The sleep itself was peaceful and uninterrupted.

Still, Bill's nonproblem has a name.

He has what is called a **delayed sleep phase syndrome,** which puts him on a different track from most of society. He has a routine that includes a late bedtime and late morning awakening. He also has a hobby that he loves, which occupies him late into the night. He has enough money to live on and enough to eat. Unlike many people who can no longer work, Bill doesn't drink or overeat.

Is his life perfect? No. He hates his disability, but he has learned to live with it and he doesn't curse his fate. He smokes cigarettes, which is always a problem, but going to bed earlier than he does wouldn't help kick that habit.

After nearly an hour with Bill, I asked, "Does going to bed late cause you any difficulty at all?" He thought for a moment, looked me in the eye, and said, "I usually have trouble getting to the Off Track Betting office in time for the race at twelve-thirty."

The fact that Bill has chosen to live the way he does—out of kilter with the conventional 24-hour day—doesn't represent an immediate threat to his health.

The problem with delayed sleep phase syndrome, however, is that the choices that people make may carry the seeds of problems further down the road. Obviously, if someone keeps Bill's hours and uses them to write the great American novel or invent a better mousetrap, there's a net social benefit. But other lifestyle choices that are expressed in delayed sleep phase syndrome may not be so constructive.

Gambling on a fixed income can become a problem. Smoking is never good for anyone's health, and it can cause poor sleep later in life even if it doesn't seem to be a problem currently. Another danger is the corrosive effects of isolation from other people, which is usually part of the equation. My recommendations to Bill and the referring doctor addressed the social issues with a summary of sleep hygiene rules. Ultimately Bill will continue to pick a pattern of sleep that will match his lifestyle choices.

The Drive to Sleep—Part of Our Elementary Humanity

Along with thirst and hunger, the drive to sleep is now recognized as one of the elementary drives for all higher animal life-forms—that is, everything more complex than a snail. In fact, as Dr. William Dement, a leading authority on sleep medicine, has pointed out, it is probably the one irresistible drive. After all, people can fast themselves to death. They can choose not to drink seawater even though they are dying of thirst. But ultimately, they cannot resist the urge to sleep. Sleep happens to you.

Indeed, sleep is a basic part of making us the people we are. It is clear that prolonged sleep deprivation has profound effects on what we think and what we do, as practitioners of torture in countries around the world have long known.

Menachem Begin, the Israeli prime minister from 1977 to 1983, was tortured by the KGB as a young man. He wrote in his memoir *Revolt* that after a period of prolonged sleep deprivation, "a haze begins to form" in the head of the prisoner. "His spirit is wearied to death, his legs are unsteady, and he has one sole desire: to sleep. . . . Anyone who has experienced this desire knows that not even hunger and thirst are comparable with it."

He said that prisoners would sign anything in return for a promise of uninterrupted sleep. "[H]aving signed, there was nothing in the world that could move them to risk again such nights and such days."

We can see that sleep deprivation strips torture victims of their dignity and their identity. It is reminiscent in that regard of what happens during another degrading human experience, withdrawal from addiction. People are willing to do anything—lie, steal from relatives, cheat—in order to be relieved of their cravings.

Of course, Begin's fellow prisoners would not have been able to foresee what would pass for entertainment in the early 21st century when Britain's Channel 4 broadcast a reality show called *Shattered* in which 10 contestants went without sleep for a week competing for a prize of £100,000.

Exhibit A: As one of them said, "It was like torture. . . . It's not every day you try to spend 180 hours without any sleep."

"Great Nature's Second Course"

Remember what Shakespeare called sleep at the beginning of this chapter, "great nature's second course." This aptly describes the role that sleep should play in our lives—something as desirable as a good day's activity. We not only *need* a good daily sleep, but we should *want* it.

We can all appreciate why the military should want to push the envelope on what the human body can withstand in the way of sleep deprivation, but as the stories about torture at the hands of the KGB—or at the hands of the British broadcast entertainment business indicate—we should not have any illusions about what sleep deprivation can do to us. It can change who we are, and it never changes us for the better.

That is why all of us owe it to ourselves, our families, our friends, and our colleagues to fix what ails our sleep. We are living longer and longer. Next time you talk with a 90-year-old, remind yourself that they needed 30 years of sleep to get there. Sleep well to live long.

3
_____

READY TO SLEEP

You would probably not say that he was sleeping the sleep of the just, unless you meant the just asleep, but it was certainly the sleep of someone who was not fooling about when he climbed into bed of a night and turned off the light.

—Douglas Adams, *The Long Dark Tea-Time of the Soul* (1988)

Much of this book is concerned with medical conditions that keep people from getting a proper night's rest. However, at the heart of all sleep problems, whether medical, behavioral, or psychological in origin, is respect for what your body wants to do, which is sleep at certain times of the day and night, and be active at others. Whatever else is going on in your life, you want to be able to put it aside at bedtime, like the fellow referred to above.

"Catch a Wave and You're Sitting on Top of the World"

I grew up listening to surf music, and while I've only windsurfed myself, I appreciated the exhilaration of catching a wave and riding it toward the beach. When the Beach Boys sang about that feeling, they could also have been referring to sleep. There are few things more satisfying than drifting off to sleep at the end of a rewarding day.

To get a good night's sleep, you have to be ready to sleep. If you think about the rhythms of your day—those circadian rhythms referred to earlier—it really is like the tides. The moon revolves around the earth once a day, the same as your daily cycle of sleeping and waking. You have your high tides and you have your low tides. The waves sometimes crash against the beach and sometimes they are relatively gentle.

Think of what surfers do to get ready to catch a wave. They study the tides. They prepare their boards. They wear a wet suit to protect them from getting too cold while they are in the water for hours and hours. At the end of all that preparation, the surfer paddles out into the ocean and bides his or her time until the right wave comes along.

Likewise, in many respects your waking life is spent preparing for sleep. You get up in the morning, shower, dress, eat breakfast, get your family and yourself out the door, spend the day at fulfilling work or other activity. If you're lucky, you have a chance to get some exercise during the day or after you leave work. You eat your evening meal, relax, read, watch TV, talk to family and friends, generally unwind, get into bed, and there you lie, sort of like that surfer, waiting for that perfect wave to come along.

Looking closely at a typical day, you may be able to chart your physical and mental highs and lows, much as an oceanographer can plot the tides. Many coincide with some pretty basic physical factors which you cannot control. Much as we might like to think that we have control over our bodies, a great deal of what we do follows inborn patterns.

Your Body Wants a Siesta

Take that midafternoon sleepiness, and that civilized custom called a siesta. Contrary to folk wisdom, this urge to lie down has little to do with sleeping off a large midday meal. Escaping the midafternoon heat? You're getting warmer. But why do some people in colder climates also crave a siesta? In fact, that midafternoon sleepiness is a temperature-related phenomenon, but it's *body* temperature. Your urge to sleep is at its highest when your body temperature takes a temporary dip after steadily increasing since early in the morning.

What genetic factor determined that our body temperature should decrease in midafternoon? We can only speculate that maybe this part of our circadian rhythm was set when our ancestors crawled back into their caves to escape the equatorial heat. In any case, it's still with us, and no modern invention like central air-conditioning has been with us long enough to reset the evolutionary clock.

Alertness, productivity, heart rates—all of them rise and fall as the circadian cycle unfolds. Your readiness to sleep at night is *normally* one more event in this daily process.

But it's not that easy, is it? All of us have problems sleeping from time to time. We lie down and sleep doesn't come. We're worried or we're happy or we've had a nice cup of coffee after a good dinner. Or maybe we wake up after a couple of hours of sound sleep. There's a noise in the night. The baby cries and after comforting him we can't get back to sleep. Maybe we've had too much to drink at dinner and after nodding off almost before we get undressed for bed, we wake up with a vengeance (and a headache) at two in the morning.

Getting Ready to Sleep

Many of us freely use the word "insomnia," which is by definition the inability to get to sleep, stay asleep, or both. While insomnia is a complex subject, which is discussed, in greater detail in Chapter 10, in many cases it stems from poor preparation for sleep. While you may have underlying medical conditions that are disturbing your sleep, at least some of your difficulties may lie in your own behavior, which is preventing you from catching the wave. For example:

- Do you drink coffee to stay awake in the afternoons or evenings?
- Do you stay in bed until the last possible moment on weekday mornings?
- Do you go to sleep after Jon Stewart's *The Daily Show,* which ends at 11:30, one night, and stay up for the Conan O'Brian show the next?
- Do you party on Friday and Saturday nights and stay in bed late on Saturday and Sunday mornings?
- Do you go out drinking with the boys, the girls, or some combination of the two regularly?

- Are you a smoker?
- Do you need a nap during the day?
- Do you actually take one?
- Do you wake up on the couch in the wee hours of the morning and drag yourself off to bed?

If you answer yes to any of these questions, there's a good chance that at least some of your sleep problems stem from your lifestyle.

The list of questions could go on and on. The point is that such behavior, whether in response to the pressures of your life, an underlying medical condition, or because of a lifestyle choice, is probably contributing to your difficulties in sleeping.

On pages 280–81 you'll find a sleep diary that is similar to what we use in our sleep center. It is easy to use, and it is one of the best tools we have for treating certain sleep problems at the least cost.

When you keep a sleep diary, you can more clearly see the problems with the amount, timing, or quality of your sleep. If the lifestyle choices are the problem, you can do something about them. You learn a great deal as you record in your sleep diary and review it with a doctor. When you average the number of hours you slept each night and look at the pattern of time to bed and wake time, you are analyzing your sleep health over that period of time. You may be very surprised to find that you average only five hours of sleep per night. Completing the diary may take some effort, but the information gained is well worth it. Recognizing and understanding the findings on a completed sleep diary can at times be all that is needed to correct the sleep disorder. And if there is a medical problem, the improved sleep will make the job of medical recovery easier.

Sleep Hygiene

Hygiene is a word we associate with avoiding the spread of disease. It seems incredible now but a century and a half ago doctors didn't even wash their hands before examining their patients.

Today, some of the biggest threats to public health around the world relate to matters of hygiene—a lack of clean water, clean blood supplies, clean food supplies, sewage treatment, sterile hypodermic needles, and so on. We take these hygiene issues as givens for good health.

Yet, very few of us really think twice about playing fast and loose with our sleeping habits. This is a big mistake.

Whether your sleep problems spring primarily from your body or your mind, your behavior as it pertains to sleep day to day—what sleep experts call sleep hygiene—has a huge influence on your overall health.

A good commonsense program of sleep hygiene is the foundation of a healthy life. It is also a critical part of treating sleep disorders, even those that require medication and technological and surgical intervention. All things considered, if you can solve your problems by changes in behavior rather than medical treatment, you are better off.

Here are the fundamentals of good sleep hygiene:

GET THE "RIGHT" AMOUNT OF SLEEP

Surfers paddle out just far enough from shore to catch the perfect wave. Good sleepers don't go to bed too early or too late. They establish a bedtime that is right for them.

Each of us needs a certain amount of sleep. Eight hours a night is a conventional benchmark, but it varies. Some people are genetically programmed for six hours of sleep and some are programmed for nine hours, but studies show that most people need about eight hours.

Studies also show that, whatever our genetic predisposition, sleep is most restful and restorative when we sleep in one relatively continuous period of time.

Many people with sleep disorders make the mistake of spending too much time in bed, either because they think they need more sleep than they do or because they operate under the impression that if they shut their eyes, sleep will come. What happens, in fact, is that their disordered sleep continues in fits and starts, and while they may end up spending the "right" nominal amount of time in bed, the sleep itself is poor in quality. The body does different things at different points during a normal night's sleep. It doesn't do them any good to just lie in bed.

REM and non-REM sleep and all the associated neurochemical processes follow a schedule. Thus, seven and a half hours of fitful sleep spread out over nine hours in bed is not as effective as seven and a half hours of continuous sleep. You will hear a great deal more about this in Chapter 15 on "The Problems of Shift Workers."

How much sleep do you need? Fill out your sleep diary for two weeks, add up the total number of hours of sleep you get, and divide by 14. This is your average daily sleep need. It should be close to eight hours. Then budget yourself for that amount of sleep plus 30 extra minutes in bed each night when you first get into bed to allow you to catch the wave.

The moon and gravity move the tide and surf; the sun sets the clock. Work with your circadian rhythms—your biological clock—by maintaining regular bedtimes and wake times, seven days a week—weekends, too! This may be harder than it sounds, because it means that you must get up at the same time each morning, even if you had trouble sleeping the night before.

The sun sets and rises at pretty much the same times, day to day, although that time changes substantially over the course of the seasons. You may want to make up for lost sleep, but the world won't cooperate because your eyes respond to sunlight and also to darkness. To get back in synch with your circadian rhythm and return to good, regular sleep may take several bad nights. It will be a little bit easier to do this if you keep a sleep diary to track your progress over the entire 24-hour day as you adjust.

LET YOUR RESPONSIBILITIES DICTATE YOUR BEDTIME

Don't forget that you have a day job. We live in a 24/7 world, but we are not 24/7 animals. Whatever part of the 24/7 world you work in, you should use the time of your greatest responsibility—work, school, taking the kids to school, and so on—to schedule your sleep.

For example, if you work nominally nine to five, but you frequently have eight o'clock business breakfasts, figure out the time you need to get up, shower, commute, and so forth to get to your appointment. Say that's 6:30. Then count back the hours you calculated as your sleep need plus 30 minutes. There. You have your bedtime. Conflict with a favorite TV show? That's why VCRs and Tivos were invented.

RELAX

You'd have to be unusual not to worry about something these days, but if you are the type of person who obsesses, you ought to do something about it. Some people find it helpful to write down their concerns or make a to-do list for the next day several hours before going to bed. But don't leave the list on your bed table or even in your bedroom where it will surely cry out for you in the middle of the night. A warm bath, some quiet music, or some relaxation exercises such as deep breathing can also be helpful.

PROTECT YOUR ENVIRONMENT

We were made to sleep in darkness. Light is a signal to your brain that it's time to leave the cave and go out to hunt for food. If we were supposed to sleep in daylight, we would have thicker eyelids.

Keep your bedroom dark. Put shades over your windows if there are streetlamps outside. Don't fall asleep with your bedside lamp on, or sleep with a night-light. Use eye shades if need be.

We were made to sleep in relative silence. Our ancestors had to put up with crickets and frogs, and our country cousins still do, but these regular noises are, if anything, soothing. We were also made to wake up to the sound of tigers roaring and other threats to life in the cave. Today, we have sirens, gunshots, and car alarms, which wake us up when there is usually no threat to life and limb. If there is no way to shut out these sounds of modernity, the next best thing is to get yourself a "white noise" machine, which emits neutral relaxing noises such as the sound of waves and otherwise obscures the din of traffic and other ambient sounds. You may also try earplugs, although this is not advisable for people with problems of the inner ear canal or hearing conditions such as tinnitus.

USE YOUR BEDROOM FOR SLEEPING
(AND FOR ONE OTHER ACTIVITY)

Do not watch television in bed. While some people find that TV watching puts them to sleep, it creates more troubles than it solves. First of all, if the show is any good, it will tempt you to stay up too late. Second, if you fall asleep with the set on, the noise will intrude on your sleep. If you start to dream about diet pills, exercise machines, or juicers, chances are you have fallen asleep and the station you were watching has gone over to "paid programming."

Don't pay your bills, work on your computer, or talk on the phone in the bedroom. In the hour before you go to sleep your body is susceptible to going either way: sleeping or staying awake. Limit your choices. If you must read in bed, and many of us must, make sure you turn off your reading light when it's time to stop. Otherwise, the light may cut your rest short by intruding on your optic nerves during a change in sleep cycles.

Make sure you have a comfortable bed and pillow. Advertisers will try to convince you that there's a magic mattress, usually at a big price above ordinary mattresses, but I don't believe it. A proper mattress should be uniformly supportive, not sagging or lumpy, but most of all it should feel right to you. Make sure you aren't allergic to your bedding; for example, if your feather pillow is making you sneeze, try something else. Above all, keep your room clean if you are prone to allergies, and even if you aren't.

Make sure that your bedroom is comfortably cool but not cold.

DON'T GO TO BED UNTIL YOU ARE FEELING SLEEPY

Many of us make the mistake of going to bed before our bodies are ready. "Lie there and sleep will come." They think somehow that they can make up for lost sleep time by spending more time in bed. Unfortunately, when the lights go out, the mind often switches on.

Putting off going to bed until the urge to sleep is really descending over you not only increases the chances of falling asleep, but reinforces the idea that bed is for sleeping. For all their wishful thinking, insomniacs, unfortunately, really associate going to bed with lying awake.

IF YOU SNOOZE, YOU LOSE

Get up at the same time every morning. Make it hard to hit the snooze button on your alarm clock by keeping it on your dresser, not on your bed table. When you leap out of bed to turn off the alarm, keep going. Don't turn back. Rising early at the same time each day establishes a baseline for a healthy sleep-wake cycle. Even good sleepers can be undermined by sleeping late. It's hard to maintain this discipline during the weekend when you want to stay up late at night and sleep later in the morning. This "social sleeping" schedule runs you into trouble, however, when you have to wake up on time to go to work on Monday. People used to say, never buy a car that was made on a Monday. I'm not sure how you were supposed to be able to tell, or what choice you had. However, while this may have been an urban legend, it reflected the suspicion that cars made on Mondays were built by workers who were still recovering from the weekend.

When you are awake, make sure you get adequate exposure to natural light. Being cut off from the cycle of daylight and darkness can throw off your biological clock. This is particularly important for older people who may not venture outside as frequently as children and adults do.

One way to set your biological clock is to spend 15 minutes in the morning sun right after you wake up.

DO NOT TAKE NAPS

Regular napping is good for narcoleptics or for people whose demanding schedules don't allow for a full night's sleep and who need a pause that refreshes during the day. Thomas Edison felt that sleep was a waste of time, although he took what Dr. James B. Maas has dubbed, "power naps" in his book *Power Sleep*.

However, for the rest of us, napping disrupts the sleep-wake cycle, particularly if we do it after dinner, which is too close to bedtime. Most insomniacs tend to nap at irregular times, which throws them further off the routine they need so badly. Problem sleepers might try substituting gentle exercise such as a walk when they have an urge to catch 40 winks.

The remaining four hygiene rules are commonsense measures for good sleep, and for good health in general.

CUT DOWN OR ELIMINATE ALCOHOL AND CAFFEINE

Never drink alcohol later than two hours before bedtime. Coffee, tea, and many soft drinks, as well as hot chocolate, all contain caffeine. Don't consume them after about 4 P.M., or lunchtime; to be safe you might even eliminate them from your diet altogether.

CUT BACK OR STOP SMOKING

Nicotine is a stimulant. If you must smoke, don't smoke within four hours of your bedtime. And never smoke in bed! On the chance that the sleep wave washes over you while you are smoking, it may be the last night you sleep, ever.

Avoid strenuous physical exertion after 6 P.M. Exercise can promote good sleep, but vigorous exercise should be taken in the morning or late afternoon. A relaxing exercise, like a low-intensity yoga, can be done before bed.

IF YOU MUST EAT BEFORE BEDTIME, EAT SPARINGLY

Food can be disruptive right before sleep; stay away from large late dinners or prebedtime snacks. When you were a child, your parents told you not to go swimming after you ate. There was a good reason for that. Just at a time when your body needs to devote its energy to swimming, it would have been sidetracked by the need to digest the food in your stomach. The same principle applies for sleep as well. You don't want your blood flow to increase at a time when your body needs to settle down. There's also the issue of weight gain by eating prior to the inactivity of sleep. Those extra calories once digested are going to remain in your body in the form of fat instead of consumed by activity as they would during the day.

Changing your diet can also cause sleep problems. Don't try a new exotic cuisine if you're having trouble sleeping. Lay off a late bowl of chocolate ice cream or chocolate in any form—it contains caffeine. If you must eat, try a light carbohydrate snack like crackers with a glass of milk. Assuming you have no other stomach problems, this might help you sleep soundly. But be careful—"*light*" *carbohydrates* doesn't mean you can eat a lot of it. A large meal of any kind will hurt your chances of getting to sleep, as well as your waistline.

RITES OF PASSAGE INTO SLEEP

Rituals play an important role in imparting a sense of stability and continuity in our lives. Even minor everyday routines have an air of ritual about them. Setting the table for an evening meal, or preparing the same comfort foods at holiday time are rituals. We develop faith in the very predictable results of those actions. Bedtime rituals can be a source of comfort and assurance that allow us to make a secure passage into sleep.

What do we do with our children in the evening to prepare them for bed? After, presumably, a nutritious meal, schoolwork, and healthy play or other activity, we bathe them, we read to them, and we may pray with them. They go to bed at the same time every night, more or less. They may not want to go to bed, but they are ready. They are never more secure. We never look stronger to them as parents, more capable, more gentle. All is right in that child's world. Thus reassured, they are ready for the wave.

Okay. It doesn't always happen that way, and even if it does, it can't last. As the kids get older, they want to stay up later. They want to watch more television and surf the Internet and talk on the phone. Catching a wave gets harder. More choices of activity at bedtime are a price we pay for growing up.

Still, some effort to re-create that sense of security, warmth, fulfillment, and respect for the biological clock is a necessary part of a good night's sleep at any stage of life.

MAKE PEACE WITH THE WORLD

Unwind early in the evening. If you take your work home with you, get it over with. Falling asleep can be almost impossible if your mind is sorting through problems, weighing decisions, and reviewing the day's activities.

Try to avoid emotionally upsetting conversations and activities before hitting the bedroom. Don't dwell on your problems or bring them to bed. Try to be on speaking terms with all the important people in your life and then some.

HAVE A BEDTIME RITUAL

You probably don't have a bedtime ritual equivalent to the one described above for children, but you might think about devising one. A ritual sends a signal to your body and your mind that it is time to settle down and fall asleep. If you consider the role of ritual in cultures around the world, whether it is the Japanese tea-drinking ritual, hanging the Christmas stockings, lighting Hanukkah candles, or facing Mecca to pray, the rituals are reassuring. We drop our childhood bedtime rituals as we get older because we don't have time, or because we "know better." But chaos at bedtime has predictable effects, too, and they are not conducive to sleep.

A ritual does not have to be a long process and can be as simple as brushing your teeth and reading for 15 minutes.

A cup of chamomile tea or another herbal tea might or might not have sedative qualities, but enjoying a cup of it can't hurt you. It contains no caffeine. The ritual of boiling the water, steeping the tea, and settling down with a warm cup in your hands has its own measure of comfort.

Take a warm bath before going to bed. Warm baths raise your body's temperature. After the bath your body cools off and this cooling is what makes you sleepy.

Catch a wave, instead of a second wind. Remember, in the hour before bedtime your body and mind can go either way. If you are distracted by non-sleep-oriented activities—another chapter of a best-selling thriller or another showing of *Spider Man* on HBO—you can upset that steady descent toward sleep. By staying up too late you are likely to revive long enough to catch a second wind instead of a wave of sleep.

Not for Insomniacs Only

Good sleep hygiene is the foundation for a good night's sleep no matter what your particular sleep problems are, be they predominantly physical in origin, subject to treatment by one or more medical specialists, or a function of your personality, your way of life, or your state of mind. The goal is approximately eight hours of restorative sleep, complete with all the stages of REM and non-REM sleep.

"Reverse Sleepology"

In this chapter we have focused on good sleep hygiene behavior and proper preparations for sleep. This presupposes that you are convinced that good sleep is possible. Some of us, however, believe that the rules do not apply to us. How do you convince a person to relax and prepare for a good night's sleep when they have "proven" to themselves over months or years that they do not sleep? This state, which is usually lumped under the heading "insomnia"—a habitual inability to get a refreshing, restorative night's sleep, assuming there is no underlying medical condition—may result from learned behavior. Instead of learning and practicing good sleep hygiene, they develop daytime and sleep habits that raise their stress levels. Treatment for this counter-productive behavior involves redirecting bedtime focus and unlearning bad habits.

Some patients do better by focusing on the other side of the coin. They already know the sleep hygiene rules and practice them for the most part. However, they do better when they direct their attention to the daytime, which prepares them for the night.

When insomnia is chronic, it continues over a longer period of time and sleeplessness begins to feed on itself. The turning point is when the effects of insomnia begin to impinge on the waking day. After battling on for a while, people begin to make allowances for the lack of sleep. They begin to react to the effects of their stressful behavior in unhealthy ways. Instead of recognizing and changing their bad habits, they curtail their normal activity instead. They make excuses. They take naps. They drink more coffee and ratchet up their daytime stress levels. Bedtime becomes a time of dread. The thought of bed and going to sleep is enough to cause some insomniacs to break out into a sweat. They get performance anxiety. When asked about the day, they complain about being tired and not satisfied with their energy level.

After a few days or weeks, it's as if someone else has taken over their bodies—someone very like themselves, to be sure, but someone who doesn't work as hard, play as hard, love as much. Instead, that person becomes, in effect, prematurely old, hypochondriacal, and self-absorbed. The sensation of being less than rested becomes a preoccupation, which then becomes an obsession.

The key to changing this downward spiral is to remember the person we were and to replace our current diminished state with the better life that person lived. It takes work, but we can redirect our focus from the sleeplessness we experience at night to making the day a more positive and easier-to-control part of our 24-hour existence.

I ask retired patients who can't sleep to picture themselves getting up early on a given day and to visualize the full day as they are living it now. Chances are, there are huge gaps in which life is not being "lived." Too much downtime. Too little activity. Too many breaks. Too much TV. What happened to the full schedule they used to have—or thought they had? The physical exercise, the mental exercise, the socializing, errands, work, projects, lively conversation, and recreation—where have they gone? Have they given up those activities because they cannot sleep? Or can they not sleep because they have given them up?

If you cannot think of enough positive things that serve to fill your day, it is probable that your daytimes are your problem, not your nights. The blame has been falling on the wrong part of the 24-hour day. This is where a new and redirected focus comes in. We try to get the person who causes insomnia by worrying about the night to plan and live a full and productive day. This is a method that involves creating good day hygiene as a first step to sleep hygiene. The day ends with a new ritual: the satisfaction that comes when any project has come to a successful conclusion, whether it is running a mile, swimming laps, pulling the last weed from the garden, or finishing a good book. You take a deep cleansing breath and relax.

We can "treat" organic sleep disorders, but only you can treat your life.

Refocusing like this is a form of cognitive therapy, which will be discussed in greater detail in Chapter 10 on insomnia. It cannot be done successfully in isolation from other forms of behavioral change, or without resolving underlying medical problems. It cannot work in the absence of good sleep hygiene. Drinking a cup of coffee or watching TV in bed will not be a constructive bedtime ritual no matter how satisfying your day has been.

This technique is not for everyone, but when it works it is very rewarding to see the improvements in sleep. Patients will usually report some improvement, along with a clearer understanding of the total 24-hour human experience. They begin to view sleep as they do proper diet and physical exercise: something that requires planning, preparation, and proper execution. If you sleep well, you will enjoy the reward of a full and productive day or wake period. If you live well and get the most out of your daytime, you will hit the pillow with a smile.

Fill Your Life with Stuff

When I go to parties where I don't know most of the guests, I try to steer the conversation away from what I do. Why? Because it seems as though *everyone* has a sleep problem, and although I love what I do, I also like to talk about other things. I try to talk about my four wonderful children, my fabulous wife who is a professional chef, wine, and especially golf, which is my own personal passion. I'd rather discuss religion and politics, which can be dangerous, than talk about sleep problems in a superficial way. It's almost impossible to offer truly useful advice without benefit of a full consultation and examination. Still, occasionally I get really lucky because I dispense simple advice that works.

I was at dinner with the father of a friend of my eldest son. He is a freelance writer and at-home dad who had a lot of trouble sleeping. He described his day to me: get the kids out of the house, work like hell all morning, make business calls in the afternoon, take care of the kids, make dinner. He enjoys his work, dealing with many clients, rather than a single boss, as he did when he had corporate jobs. He has very close relationships with all his children.

What was missing from his existence was a good deal of the connective tissue that holds the days of most people together. Commuting. Lunch with colleagues. Meetings. Couple that with the uncertainties and distractions of almost any self-employed, home-based business and you come up with a textbook case of insomnia. Anxiety. Speculation. Worry. Isolation. Too much brain and not enough to occupy it. This is particularly the case when someone "thinks" for a living, which writers do. They need a way to turn off the continual flow of words and ideas through their heads. My advice to him was, "Fill your days with 'stuff.' Work in the garden, join a gym, cook more elaborate meals."

There was nothing profound about any of this. It's good commonsensical advice for anyone. However, many of us lack the discipline to act sensibly. In this case, it worked quite well. We have become quite good friends since then. Now when we meet socially we talk about our children, food and wine, politics and religion, and even golf, which he doesn't play, but he likes the idea of it.

Not every moment of our day has to be entertaining or profound. But if we spend the vast majority of time absorbed in our waking activities, we will make our nighttimes better.

As Leonardo da Vinci put it, "A well-spent day brings happy sleep."

4

GOOD DAYS, BAD DAYS

Sleeping is no mean art: for its sake one must stay awake all day.

—Friedrich Nietzche

Nietzche may have been a controversial figure but he wasn't stupid. All would agree that he sensed the delicacy of the relationship between daytime wakefulness and nighttime sleep. Today, we pay strict attention to days as an indicator of what is going on at night. What we call "excessive daytime sleepiness" is a sure sign that something is wrong.

POP QUIZ
EPWORTH SLEEPINESS SCALE*

How likely are you to doze off or fall asleep in the following situations, in contrast with feeling just tired? (Even if you have not done some of these things recently, try to consider how they tend to affect you.) Use the following scale to choose the most appropriate number for each situation:

0 = would never doze
1 = slight chance of dozing
2 = moderate chance of dozing
3 = high chance of dozing

Situation	Chance of Dozing
Sitting and reading	_____
Watching TV	_____
Sitting, inactive in a public place (e.g., a theater or meeting)	_____
As a passenger in a car for an hour without a break	_____
Lying down to rest in the afternoon when circumstances permit	_____
Sitting and talking to someone	_____
Sitting quietly after a lunch without alcohol	_____
In a car, while stopped for a few minutes in the traffic	_____
TOTAL	_____

A score of nine or more indicates potentially pathologic sleepiness that should be evaluated by a sleep physician.

*This test was developed by Dr. Murray Johns at Epworth Hospital in Melbourne, Australia in 1991 © 1991–1997.

The test above is called the Epworth Sleepiness Scale. Like so much of sleep medicine, or all preventative medicine for that matter, it puts patients on the front lines of their own treatment. Initial suspicion of a sleep disorder is often *subjective;* that is, it depends on the patient's own perceptions of his or her condition, and not on tests we do in a laboratory, measuring brain waves and so forth.

If you measure nine or more on the Epworth Scale, your problem may be serious, and not temporary. Instead, you may have an underlying medical or sleep disorder that is drastically compromising your quality of life and seriously undermining your health in both the short and long term. A doctor would call what you have EDS—excessive daytime sleepiness.

Although figures vary, EDS is common and occurs in 5–30 percent of the general population. The majority of patients who come to our sleep center have EDS. Hypersomnia is increased sleepiness during the day or extended sleepiness during the night and is often used to describe the daytime part of EDS. EDS is a problem that is very different from insomnia, although patients often confuse the two. People who suffer from some form of insomnia—those whose chief complaint is that they can't sleep at night—also complain of EDS. However, for the most part they focus more on the night symptoms. They usually don't pay as much attention to their daytime problems, even though their daytime performance may be less than optimal. They often try to treat their nighttime problems themselves. They buy more self-help books than other people, drink more herbal tea, and meditate. When you consider that almost as many people try to treat their sleeplessness with alcohol as use medication, you can appreciate how many people try to deal with insomnia on their own. For those with insomnia who do come to the sleep center we have a dedicated insomnia program. I will discuss insomnia in detail in Chapter 10.

EDS patients are another matter. They cannot live their lives. As John Cunningham, the technical director of our lab, puts it, "These patients don't even recognize when they are sleepy, or they think that it is normal." As a result, EDS, like most other sleep disorders, is underreported. Almost any cessation of activity is enough to trigger sleep onset and, as a result, EDS is a frequent cause of traffic accidents, poor evaluations at work, and computer screens that look like this:

eeeeeeeeeeeeeeeeeeeeeeeeeeeeeeeeeeeeeeeeeeeeeeeeeeeeeeeeeeeeee
eeeeeee

eeeeeeeeeeeeeeeeeeeeeeeeeeeeeeeeeeeeeeeeeeeeeeeeeeeeeeeeeeeeeeeeeee
eeeeeee
eeeeeeeeeeeeeeeeeeeeeeeeeeeeeeeeeeeeeeeeeeeeeeeeeeeeeeeeeeeeeeeeeee
eeeeeee
eeeeeeeeeeeeeeeeeeeeeeeeeeeeeeeeeeeeeeeeeeeeeeeeeeeeeeeeeeeeeeeeeee
eeeeeee

When this happens, you don't have to know much about physiology to know that there's something wrong.

Many of us only know we've had a good day when it's over and we have time to reflect. We bounced out of bed in the morning (or whenever we got out of bed—it's not the same for everyone), showered, dressed, went to work or school where we lost ourselves in eight sustained hours of rewarding activity, left, ate dinner with family or friends or spent the evening doing something to unwind. If we were really good, we took time for some exercise.

If you were having substantially more good days than bad days, you probably wouldn't be reading this book at all. People with EDS don't have good days. Their sleepiness casts a pall over all their other activities. To paraphrase President John F. Kennedy, an ebbing tide lowers all boats.

Normal and Abnormal Sleepiness

Sleepiness is a natural part of your day. That is, your *24-hour* day. Normally, sleepiness peaks at bedtime and continues through the sleep period. If it overwhelms us during the day, there's something wrong.

We all have occasional daytime sleepiness, but for the most part this is a result of temporary sleep deficit, such as when there's a new baby at home or a sick child or you've been burning the candle at both ends. Your problem is an absence of sleep. This can become a longer-term problem if you develop bad sleep habits as a result, but sleep deficit is often a behavioral issue that can be reversed by changing the behavior, as explained in the previous chapter.

When severe, EDS patients have an irresistible urge to sleep. When that urge overtakes them, it can be almost intoxicating, and certainly seems preferable to fighting to stay awake. This is not a lack of concentration or boredom or yawning. This is surrender. The brain is demanding sleep and has the ability to independently flip the master switch to a sleep state. EDS is most often caused by sleep deprivation or insufficiency. Other causes include not only sleep disorders but injuries, medications, and so forth.

Untreated **obstructive sleep apnea,** which involves cessation of breathing due to blockage of the windpipe during sleep; **narcolepsy,** which results from a faulty switch between waking and sleep; and **restless legs syndrome,** which produces uncomfortable sensations in the legs that can only be relieved by voluntary movement, are the sleep disorders responsible for most cases of excessive sleepiness evaluated and diagnosed at sleep centers.

Not all EDS is the same. Variations in the daytime symptoms may point to a specific underlying sleep disorder. In the case of obvious sleep apnea the history and physical examination are highly predictive.

Symptoms of Sleep Apnea	
Daytime symptoms	Nighttime symptoms
EDS	Loud snoring, choking
Naps, too long and unrefreshing	Breathing stops
Personality change	Sitting up, fighting for sleep
Morning headaches	Abnormal motor movements
Inability to concentrate	Esophageal reflux
Impotence	Frequent urination
	Profuse sweating

Narcolepsy and restless leg syndrome both have very specific daytime signs and symptoms in addition to EDS and when full-blown are fairly easy to diagnose. Each of these disorders will be dealt with in later chapters.

Occasionally, problems unrelated to sleep may be discovered at sleep centers when general practitioners refer patients who have symptoms they attribute to EDS. Multiple sclerosis, cancer, hypothyroidism, chronic infections, and withdrawal from alcohol or any substance can leave patients exhausted, but not sleepy in the sense that we use it here. Brain tumors, trauma, and degenerative diseases such as Parkinson's disease can cause EDS. We do not treat these conditions at a sleep center, per se, but we can direct the care to one of our multispecialty consultants or other doctors after we have eliminated a diagnosis of sleep disorder.

Medication, too, can be a problem. Valium-like antianxiety drugs and older, over-the-counter antihistamines have "sedative" effects. Read the warnings on the packaging—they say don't drive or operate heavy machinery. Once again, staying true to the recurrent theme of this book, sleep doctors must also consider the patient as a 24-hour-per-day complex being. We work with your other doctors, not independently of them.

WORDS CONFUSE DIAGNOSIS

Part of the problem is language. Most patients (and many health care providers) lack the vocabulary to describe symptoms accurately. Thus, their illness is mistakenly linked with a sleep disorder when it is really part of another condition.

Distinctions should be made among fatigue, simple tiredness, depression, and excessive daytime sleepiness. The word "fatigue" is often used interchangeably with these other complaints and conditions, but they are not the same. Fatigue can be associated not with sleepiness but with weariness, lack of energy, tiredness or weakness, especially that associated with aches and pains in the joints and muscles. Fatigue does not make you sleepy; it makes you miserable. You may not be sharp and alert, but neither are you really tired. You don't have an irresistible urge to shut your eyes and drift off. You have a strong desire for relief from the discomfort called fatigue. You wish you could get some sleep to get away from the feeling, not necessarily because you need the sleep itself. The confusion that results is enough to occasionally send treatment off on an entirely wrong track.

Simple tiredness is occasionally experienced by most people and may be related generally to activity level and partially to our circadian rhythm changes at certain periods during the day. Depressed patients will often have complaints of insomnia, inability or unwillingness to get out of bed, or an urge to nap to ease the depression.

The Epworth Scale presented at the beginning of this chapter is very useful as the first line of defense for separating sleep disorders from other problems. However, the gold standard for actually measuring sleepiness is called the multiple sleep latency test (MSLT). This is the test that helps us measure whether you are sleepy enough to be a danger to yourself and to others every time you sit behind the wheel of your car.

During your usual wake time, which is not the same for everybody, electrodes are attached to various parts of your head and body, which are connected to video monitors in another room. Then you lie down. You shut your eyes. During five separate nap opportunities over the next eight to nine hours, your tendency to sleep is measured in minutes and averaged out. If you begin to fall asleep in less than five minutes, you have a severe, pathologic sleep tendency. Five to 10 minutes is deemed mildly to moderately abnormal, and more than 10 is not deemed to be a problem at all. During the MSLT we also look for REM sleep in order to help us make a diagnosis of disorders such as narcolepsy. This is discussed more in Chapter 8, on narcolepsy.

For patients with pathologic sleepiness, we advise them not to drive and to use caution in the workplace until they are fully treated. This applies to operating heavy machinery and to other jobs as well. People who fall asleep at their desks are less productive than their alert colleagues.

There is good news, however. Sleepiness is usually a reversible state, like hunger and thirst. Sleepiness associated with sleep deprivation can be reversed by sleeping. Excessive daytime sleepiness can be reversed by treating the underlying sleep disorder or medical cause, and when that cause is treated, the overwhelming urge to sleep can go away.

GOLD STANDARD IN ACTION

Sometimes you can have sleep apnea without experiencing daytime sleepiness, although I happen to think that it's just a matter of time before EDS is noticed if the apnea is left untreated. One of my patients was a bus driver who was diagnosed with apnea without ever exhibiting EDS. His treatment was initiated at the urging of his wife, who hated watching and listening to him sleep. He started using a CPAP machine and went on a weight loss and general conditioning program, which he worked at diligently.

However, the diagnosis and treatment for apnea were enough to ring alarm bells in the transit medical department. He had, in effect, to be pronounced free of daytime sleepiness before he could be cleared for his normal duties. The medical officers acted responsibly.

I arranged for an MSLT. He passed with flying colors, and my report to the medical authority was enough to help get him back on the job. In essence, it said that he was fully alert during his waking hours and not a threat to his passengers, other drivers, pedestrians, or himself.

For the Birds

As a matter of law all men and women are supposedly created equal. But of course we are born with substantial differences. One of these is how we are programmed to sleep. Simply put, some of us are "day" people and some of us are "night" people. This is not just an old wives' tale, or old husbands' tale for that matter. Neither is it largely a question of how we choose to live our lives. Rather, there are distinct differences in the way we are hardwired to cope with the 24-hour day.

How can we tell who is which? By the time we reach adulthood, the distinction has pretty well sorted itself out. Genetics has a tremendous influence on our choice of occupation and general lifestyle. Day people, who include most of us, opt for a nine-to-five occupation. You can find night people working the dinner shift at restaurants or the "graveyard shift" at major daily newspapers. You can find them on both sides of the bar at your local tavern or staffing the emergency room at night at your hospital.

It's safe to say that major parts of our culture would not exist as we know them if there weren't this physiological dichotomy. There was a very funny parody a number of years ago of *Mr. Rogers' Neighborhood* in which Mr. Rogers has a jazz musician as a guest on his show. Needless to say, the musician has not been to sleep after working the night before and is groggy and uncomprehending when his host questions him about his art for the audience of preschool children.

Would we have jazz if there were no night people?

Logically, night people are often referred to as owls, while day people are called larks. Night people or owls are shown to have slightly higher rates of some of the problems we associate with inadequate sleep. I would say that this is likely to be a function of the genetic imprint that makes them owls, coupled with the stresses of being night people in a world that is skewed in favor of the day people. Just as being left-handed in a right-handed world is more stressful than being right-handed, night people living in a day-oriented world must make adjustments that often cut into their sleep. Night shift workers find it more challenging to be parents, for example, and have to burn their own candle at both ends to some extent to maintain what they think is a healthy family life. As we will see in Chapter 15, this is not true.

This leads me to a third category of bird for our aviary, which is not uniquely American, but given the prevalence of swing shifts, overtime, sleep-be-damned 12-hour working days, and just-in-time inventory in this country, we can proudly recognize it as our own—the eagle. The eagle is determined to conquer the limits of his or her own circadian rhythms. These are the swing shift workers, the long-distance truckers, the overtime gluttons. They are also highly paid professionals for whom time is money, *lots* of money: investment bankers, deal makers, management consultants, and high-level computer programmers.

Ann Winblad, venture capitalist and former girlfriend of Bill Gates, among the world's richest men, told a journalist at the height of the Internet boom, "If you don't work 12 hours a day, you're behind. If you don't read 100 trade magazines, don't check your email, don't return somebody's call, or don't go to a developer event, you're behind. Either you're committed or you're not." That from one of the people who brought us the way of life behind the term "24/7." No wonder the dot-com boom fell apart—the people who built it collapsed from exhaustion.

The all-time number one eagle may have been a Wall Street lawyer during the go-go days of the 1980s who worked 24 hours in New York and then got on a plane for a meeting in Los Angeles, working the whole way as the time zones changed, so that he could bill more than 24 hours in a single calendar day. Someone should tell him that the oxygen content of air on an airplane is significantly lower than it is on the ground, which means that if his brain needed a full dose of oxygen to complete his task he may have come up a little short on that particular project. Maybe he should charge his clients only 75 percent of his fee for the work he does on a plane.

We Can't All Be Eagles

Not everyone can be an eagle, and not everyone should want to be. Venture capitalists and corporate lawyers are very well paid for their work, but most of us earn a salary and while there may be a pay differential for working the night shift, it may not be worth the cost in diminished quality of life or health. Being a night person may be a physiological fact of life for some of us. Fortunately, there are outlets for such people in our economy, and particularly where I practice, the "city that doesn't sleep." But for those people physiologically inclined to to be night owls, there are health consequences. The night owl must manage his or her life carefully.

FLY BY DAY OR FLY BY NIGHT?

HOW THE LARK AND OWL DIFFER OVER 24 HOURS

	3 AM	5	7	9	11	12–1 PM	3	5	7	9	11	12 AM–1 AM
L A R K	Lowest heart rate, middle of sleep, melatonin peaks, low temp		Alarm optional, breakfast favorite meal, caffeine not critical	"Wired," talkative, good time for exercise	Got to work on time, peak heart rate about 11 AM, peak alertness about 12 noon	Likes day shift, AM projects	Temp peaks about 2:30, then falls		Starting to feel the day, tired	Winding down	Surf's up: catching the wave of sleep	More jet lag than owls going westward
	NIGHT				DAY						NIGHT	
TIME	3 AM	5	7	9	11	12–1 PM	3	5	7	9	11	12 AM–1 AM
O W L	Can adjust to night shift or rotating shift	Alarm and bucket of cold water to wake up, lowest heart rate, middle of sleep, melatonin peaks, low temp	Tired, quiet, grumpy even, gets up too late to eat or exercise, got to get to work	Often late to work, slow start, needs a pot of coffee to get going		Drinks coffee or caffeinated beverage with lunch	Nap if possible		Peak activity, start PM projects, peak alertness, peak heart rate about 6 PM	Temp peaks, then falls, continues to feel energized, best meal dinner	Best work, energized after entertaining and late business dinner. PM projects	Catches this later wave of sleep, adjustment easier than larks to jet lag, especially when going west
	NIGHT			DAY							NIGHT	

How different are night owls from larks? As you can see from the time line, night owls' bodies do the same things that larks' do; they just do them on a different schedule. Those differences are hardwired into their physical constitutions. A night owl will never be quite as good at a nine-to-five job as a lark, and vice versa. As long as they adapt to their pre-programmed time clocks and follow good hygiene measures, EDS (or ENS for the night shift worker) should not be a problem.

Eagles, or larks and owls for that matter, who constantly fly against the winds of their internal time-clock will develop EDS. Thomas Edison said, "Sleep is an acquired habit. Cells don't sleep. Fish swim in the water all night. Even a horse doesn't sleep. A man doesn't need any sleep." He was referring specifically to his need to fill every waking and sleeping moment with revolutionary inventions some of which would allow him to burn the midnight bulb and work throughout the night. But he was Thomas Edison. The rest of us who lack his particular bird's-eye view of the world need a more structured existence. We need to perch on a regular schedule in order to fly in our own way.

5

SNORING—NOT A LAUGHING MATTER

This self-examination, one of several discussed in this chapter, is best done while brushing your teeth.

   Look directly into the mirror, open your mouth, and stick out your tongue. What do you see?

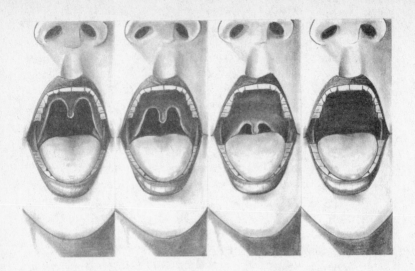

The further you get to the right of the scale, the more likely you are to snore, and the worse your snoring is likely to be for you.

Snoring Izzzzzzzzzzzzzzzz Not a Laughing Matter

If you grew up as I did watching the Three Stooges on TV, you may remember the scene where they are lying in bed, each snoring in a different tone. Classic (well, classic for the Three Stooges). In fact, snoring has long been a staple of television comedy. In almost every family there's someone who snores, and everyone else makes fun of them for it.

In my family, Grandpa complained that Grandma snored, although she denied it, and my father-in-law, a firefighter, used to complain about his buddies in the barracks at his engine company. All this was cute family gossip, always good for a laugh. But of course, the rest of us didn't have to live with the noise.

How little we knew. Today, when I think of those Three Stooges episodes, as well as Bugs Bunny and other cartoons, I feel a bit the way I do when I watch old movies where people smoke cigarettes and swill martinis without any concern for their health. Snoring was to comedy what liquor and cigarettes were to sophistication. Today, excessive smoking and boozing are movie shorthand for bad character or at least confusion and rebellion. When will snoring raise cries of alarm?

Snoring is anything but funny. It's dangerous. The decibel levels from snoring can be high enough to cause damage to the human ear. If your snoring Uncle Mike were factory machinery, according to OSHA (Occupational Safety and Health Administration) standards he'd have to be shut down or refitted. Think about that. Think what Aunt Sadie has to put up with. Imagine your spouse saying, "Honey, the government is going to shut you down until you stop snoring."

This isn't comedy. If you or your bed partner snores, you should know that snoring has been linked to serious medical problems for both of you. Approximately 20 percent of the general population snore, rising to as much as 60 percent of men over age 40. And what is it doing to them? The table below summarizes the spectrum of disorders associated with snoring, which at the sleep center we refer to as part of a larger group of conditions known as **sleep-disordered breathing** ranging from simple snoring to sleep apnea.

Not everyone who snores has sleep apnea, but most people who have sleep apnea snore. Apnea means that breathing stops. For obstructive sleep apnea, which is the kind we deal with most often, this is due to closure or blockage of the air passage. To help a patient visualize what happens, I compare this blockage during sleep to a cork suddenly blocking the opening in a bottle. Another condition, **hypopnea**, refers to incomplete blockage. Air movement decreases, but doesn't stop. Apnea and hypopnea are discussed in Chapter 6.

Snoring and Sleep Disordered Breathing		
Simple snoring	Complicated snoring	Sleep apnea
Vibration of tissue anywhere along the airway	For example upper airway resistance syndrome	Complete blockage or cessation of breathing repeatedly during sleep
May be associated with medical problems such as high blood pressure and obesity	Strong association with medical problems, disturbed sleep, and excessive daytime sleepiness (EDS)	Associated with hypertension, heart disease, diabetes, and obesity

SNORING: Why We Don't Seek Treatment

Picture yourself riding on a crowded bus or train. The man next to you starts to cough . . . and cough . . . and cough. How do you react? You shield your face with your newspaper. You turn or lean away from him. People around you start to move away both out of fear of "catching something" or out of disgust—the wetter the cough, the worse the sound. You can bet that none of this is lost on Mr. Cough. He is embarrassed by the effect he is having on people around him and would like to disappear. When he gets to work, his colleagues hear and see him cough. They ask him, "Have you been to the doctor?" They are concerned not only that he may have a serious respiratory illness but that they may get sick, too. The same kind of thing will take place at home. All of these expressions of concern and pressures make it far more likely that Mr. Cough will go to the doctor.

What does this have to do with snoring? Well, think of all the pressures Mr. Cough is under. He hears himself cough. He feels it. He accumulates phlegm in his throat. He sees the people around him turning away. His colleagues and family tell him to go to the doctor. He knows that the cough may indicate an infection or something more serious.

Now compare all of that personal and social pressure with what Mr. Snore goes through. Mr. Snore makes more noise than his cousin Mr. Cough, but he sleeps through it and doesn't know how bad it is until someone tells him. Strangers never hear him snore, unless he's lucky enough to catch a few winks on the train on the way to work. When he gets to work, his colleagues won't know he has a problem since he will be (more or less) awake. If he dozes off in a $100 seat at a Broadway show, people may tap him on the shoulder or his wife or date will elbow him in the ribs, but since there's no danger of contagion, they usually don't change seats.

Snoring affects only a select group beyond the individual snorer, mainly the witnesses. As a result there is a different type of reinforcement for the idea of medical care, something we term socially unacceptable noise. If Mr. Snore lives alone, he may be oblivious to his problem. There's an old philosophical question: If a tree falls in a forest and no one is around to hear it, does it make any noise? In the sleep business, the answer is easy: Even if there's no one around to hear you sawing logs, it's still a symptom of some very common conditions with the potential for great harm.

Surprisingly the witness and others may also be in danger. If our snorer has a spouse or bed partner or roommate, they will generally not raise any alarms about potential harm to their own physical health, as would be the case with persistent coughing. The bed partner will suffer the behavior and report it with some of the usual descriptive figures of speech: "You snored like a bear," or "The windows were rattling." More troubling, they may say, "I slept on the couch." Worse still, they may say, "I can't take it anymore. I'm calling a lawyer." But the problem is unlikely to make it as far as a doctor's office. Snoring is contagious and dangerous, but it's not the condition itself that "infects" your partner. What the bed partner catches is sleeplessness. In fact, bed partners of snorers suffer almost as much as snorers themselves and thus are one of the best predictors of a dangerous sleep disorder.

Partners of snorers are shown to have their sleep interrupted 21 times a night, versus 27 for the snorer. This level of sleep interruption is dangerous when you consider the consequences of sleep deprivation during the day. These secondhand snoring victims can fall asleep while driving or operating machinery. The people they damage when they doze off could be victims of *thirdhand* snoring.

The noise may also make their bed partners deaf—Canadian studies have shown that bed partners of snorers have a substantial incidence of partial deafness in the ear that faces their snoring bedmate. Beyond that there are psychological conditions such as depression, anxiety, and so forth that can be caused or exacerbated by sleep deprivation.

Not all snoring reaches the bed partner's threshold of pain. Occasionally it can be soothing. I once treated a man for snoring whose wife then came to me to treat her for insomnia. She was so accustomed to sleeping through his snoring that she couldn't get used to the peace and quiet.

Waking Up to the Dangers of Snoring

In the past, if snorers did make appointments with doctors about their condition, the doctor probably simply prescribed earplugs for the complaining spouse.

However, that doesn't mean that people *didn't* go to the doctor for snoring-related conditions. They went to the doctor for things like hypertension, diabetes, heart disease, and vascular disease, all of which might well have been connected to their snoring and apnea, but no one knew it.

That is changing. It is changing for you and your loved ones right now because you are reading this book. A visit to your family doctor for treatment of these and many more conditions will soon include routine questions about your sleeping habits. Most doctors advise patients with conditions like hypertension and diabetes to lay off greasy burgers, fries, and soft drinks and to get more exercise. Now, thanks to organizations like the National Heart, Lung and Blood Institute

(NHLBI, formerly the NIH) the National Sleep Foundation, the American Academy of Sleep Medicine, and sleep societies worldwide, they may also tell you to change the way you sleep.

Nighttime is a third of your life. It should not be ignored. If you have an untreated sleep disorder, your body is suffering and you are paying the price.

The Anatomy of Snoring

Snoring is a by-product of both the "hardware" and "software" of your face and upper airways. The hardware consists of a set of bones in our face, the upper part or maxilla on the top and mandible on the bottom. These form a rigid box that houses the software—the soft tissues in the nose and throat, which include the tongue, the uvula, and the tonsils.

Snoring is the vibration of those tissues along the path from the nose to the back of the throat. Even if you have never heard yourself snore, as is likely, you probably know how to make a snoring sound. Chances are you've pretended to be asleep or tried to show someone how boring you think they are by making a snoring sound. You pressed your tongue over the back of your throat and inhaled. The effect is a convincing snoring sound.

The main structures involved when you make snoring noises are the inside and back part of the nose, called the nasopharynx, the oropharynx which includes the back of the tongue, tonsils and uvula—the fleshy centerpiece extension of the soft palate that hangs down in the back of your mouth—and the base of the tongue near the hypopharynx. All are part of the upper airway, through which air must flow.

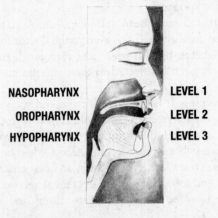

NASOPHARYNX   LEVEL 1

OROPHARYNX   LEVEL 2

HYPOPHARYNX   LEVEL 3

It is this vital pathway that is involved in both snoring and obstruction of airflow, or apnea. Snoring is a vibration of the soft tissues as the air passes over them.

Snoring is related closely to blockage, since swollen tissues or large tissues are more likely to vibrate or rattle against the nearby air tubes. A critical amount of swelling or enlargement or anything that makes the bottleneck narrower will contribute to some closure, or apnea. Any narrowing in the upper airways makes the job of getting air to your lungs that much more difficult. Think of breathing in through a cocktail straw compared with breathing through a large soda straw. The chest works harder to suck the air into the lungs. In the process, the soft tissues collapse and vibrate.

If you want to see what happens to your airways when you snore or completely block airflow, as in apnea, get out the vacuum cleaner. The vacuum motor represents the chest wall, which pulls in air as it expands. The hose is equivalent to the three divisions of the pharynx (see diagram on page 66). The front attachment where the dirt and the air enter corresponds to the nose and mouth.

Turn on the machine. It is now inhaling—a vacuum cleaner doesn't need to exhale in the same way a person does, obviously. Sounds nice and even. The only sounds are the motor and the rush of air. Now, place your hand over the end of the hose. The sound changes. It may emit a whistle, or a snorting noise. If you block the intake completely for a few seconds, not only will you feel your skin get sucked in but the vacuum hose will start to collapse on itself. When you're vacuuming, if you try to pick up something that's too big to go in, and the object gets stuck in the hose, it can sound quite literally like snoring. In reality the mechanism of snoring is much more complicated although this simplified model helps us visualize the end result: blockage or narrowing of the airway.

All of these sounds and physical actions have their counterparts in your nighttime breathing. In the throat the noise starts when the tissues such as the uvula and the tongue relax during sleep, narrowing or blocking the airways. Why are they doing this? Maybe you have gained weight and some of it has gone to your neck. Maybe Mom or Dad snored and you inherited their facial structure and large palate or tongue. Maybe you have something growing in there that shouldn't be. Or maybe your allergies are causing postnasal drip and when you lie down and put your head back on the pillow, the swelling and mucus block the back of your throat. Most important, unlike the vacuum hose the walls of the airway or pharynx muscles relax during sleep and so are more prone to collapse.

If you are vacuuming and something gets stuck in the attachment, you'd clear it out because not only is the noise awful but the carpet will take longer to clean because of the reduced suction force. In the long run, too, you'd burn out the motor.

All too often, nighttime airway blockage cannot be easily or quickly reversed. You don't act to clean out the attachment on the spot. Night after night you ignore it or don't know about it, which means, like the vacuum cleaner, your chest has to work too hard to draw in the requisite amount of air.

If the apnea or blockage is severe, it causes a shortage of oxygen. You might as well be sleeping with a bag over your head. Instead of inhaling the amount of air you need, all that soft throat tissue is collapsing, which isn't very good for it, either. Over a period of time, these tissues will swell and lose their natural resiliency.

We will review the impact of apnea on your body in the next chapter. For now, however, snoring has its own set of problems. Think about what all that vibration is doing to your body! Think about the last time you heard unusual noise or felt vibration in a car or other piece of expensive equipment. You know from experience that if you ignore it, it will lead to trouble. It is the same with all-night vibration and noise in your head.

Bad Vibrations

How much physical damage does the vibration from snoring do to your body? The science is unfolding, but the simple answer is "a whole lot."

HEARING

Research on guinea pigs shows that exposure to long-term whole-body vibration damages the tissues of the inner ear. The stronger the vibration and the closer the source, the greater the damage. Study authors concluded: "The results . . . demonstrate the harmful effect of mechanical vibration on the inner ear. According to the observed pattern of damage, one can expect an increasing hearing impairment in the low and medium frequency range in persons exposed to whole-body vibration."

Don't forget, your ears are right next to your throat! Think Uncle Eugene is going deaf just because he's getting old? Maybe he snores!

Vibration can damage your blood vessels. A group of researchers in Wisconsin studied the effects of localized vibration on rat tails, which contain arteries and nerves similar to those in the human hand. The tails were selectively vibrated for one or nine days. One four-hour session injured **endothelial** cells, which line the veins and arteries. Vibration for nine days caused loss and thinning of these cells, and activation of platelets coating the exposed subendothelial tissue. The platelets came loose and built up in blood vessels where they don't belong. Buildup of platelets and the narrowing of blood vessels is one factor known to increase your chances of heart blockage and stroke. Another study using laser Doppler surface recording showed that even five minutes of vibration significantly diminished tissue-blood perfusion, which is the ability of the blood to supply tissues with oxygen and other nutrients.

NERVES

Jobs in which workers receive heavy exposure to vibration and noise have been shown to damage the nervous system in ways that impair cardiovascular functions. Over time, this exposure hurts the physical performance of their jobs. That is one of the reasons there are legal limits on the decibel level of noise in the workplace. Levels that exceed these limits may be shut down. Yet, some snorers produce noise that exceeds the levels that would require that their workplace be closed.

Nerve damage from snoring can also hurt your airways. As you know from your vacuum cleaner, the health of the machine depends on the free flow of air; the tube collapses when obstructed. Likewise, the health of your upper airways depends on the free flow of air in and out. There's a balance between the pressure on the tissues of your airway when you are inhaling and action of the muscles that expand and contract the lungs. During sleep that action happens automatically, controlled by the nervous system.

Nerve endings in the pharyngeal mucosa—the mucous membranes that line the pharynx—act like traffic signals for directing the movement of the airway and communicating with the brain, depending whether you are inhaling or exhaling. As you will see in the detailed discussion of sleep apnea in the next chapter, the control mechanism is very sophisticated and literally saves you from choking to death hundreds of times a night.

However, chronic vibration of the tissues around these nerve endings, as when you are snoring, can disturb and damage them. Studies have shown that most patients with heavy snoring and respiratory disturbance had signs of lesions in the nerve tissues of the pharynx. These lesions may contribute to the collapse of upper airway.

Things to Look Out For

Usually, you can't hear yourself snore. So how do you tell if you're doing it or not? Here are some physical, medical, and environmental factors you and your doctor can look for that are likely to increase the likelihood that you will snore:

External. Obesity, or a neck that is too large. If your shirt collars are tighter than they used to be, you may be a snorer.

Facial structure: narrow or small nose, small lower jaw

Internal. Tissue swelling, nasal polyps, severe allergic swelling in the nose and throat

Large palate, tongue, tonsils, adenoids

Medical conditions that weaken the throat muscles. Stroke, Parkinson's disease

Lifestyle. Carbohydrate-heavy diet, exposure to inhaled allergens or respiratory irritants such as paints and solvents, use of tobacco, alcohol or medicines that relax or sedate

Behaviorial. Excessive sleepiness during the day. This is the canary in the coal mine; the surest indication that something is going wrong at night.

Are You a Violin or a Cello?

The volume of noise you make when you snore, and the level of vibration you inflict on your body and the ears of your bed partner, depends to a great extent on the way you are built. Another way to picture it is to think of your upper airway as a cello or a violin. The air going across the soft tissues of your throat is like a bow going back and forth across the strings. The resulting vibration resonates in the interior of the "instrument," which, depending on the size and shape, will produce a different level of noise. Some people are built like violins, some are built like cellos, and some are built like other members of the string family of instruments.

The bones of your face may provide you with ample room to breathe. If, however, that rigid box is narrower, when combined with malleable soft tissues in the relaxation of sleep, it may be more likely to produce that awful noise. Unfortunately, regardless of whether you are built more like a violin or a cello, the sound it makes will have more in common with someone who is just taking up the instrument than with Isaac Stern or Yo-Yo Ma. If I could snore Mozart, I probably would.

You can establish for yourself whether you are more or less prone to snoring.

Self-examination

Step 1: Start with the general shape of your face.

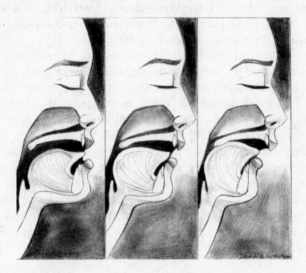

Either get someone to photograph you in profile or stand in front of your bathroom mirror with a hand mirror held off to the side and at an angle so it reflects your face from the side.

To evaluate the tendency to snore, I look for the three basic shapes of the lower jaw, as shown.

Because the tongue sits in and is attached to the inside of the lower jaw, the smaller and farther back the jaw sits, the greater the chance that the tongue can fall across the back of the throat and block the breathing passage when you sleep. Dentists often identify the backward position of the jaw in patients with an overbite or malocclusion.

This is especially true when you are lying on your back during dream or REM sleep when your body is paralyzed with atonia (see Chapter 2) and the muscles in your tongue are also relaxed.

The tongue, we know, helps us to speak and to swallow our food. However, what is not so obvious is that it helps us move air and breathe. This function becomes much more difficult if the shape of the jaw, mouth cavity, or tongue is out of proportion with the general shape of the face. For example, people with very large tongues, which occurs with a condition called macroglossia and is seen in people with growth hormone disorders, have a particular problem. This could be a good thing, if, say, you are Gene Simmons, singer for the rock band KISS, whose trademark is an oversized tongue, which he sticks out frequently when he is performing. I am, however, concerned about whether or not the large tongue affects his sleeping.

Even those with normal-sized tongues are in trouble if their tongues are out of proportion to the size of the box or bones in which the tongue is housed. During sleep, when the tongue muscle is not being used to speak or swallow, it may move against the back of the breathing space. If you snore, do the following (do not do it if you have a jaw problem like TMJ, or a locking jaw):

While sitting up with your mouth slightly open, gently inhale three times while purposely trying to snore. In the middle of the third inhalation, jut your jaw forward as far as it will comfortably go. If the snoring becomes less intense or disappears, you will know firsthand how important the tongue and lower jaw are to your airway. This simple exercise is not an accurate test for a medical condition and only helps you understand how the tongue alters the airway.

Step 2: Take another look at the diagram presented on page 73 (depicted again here on the top panel) along with the corresponding side view (bottom panel).

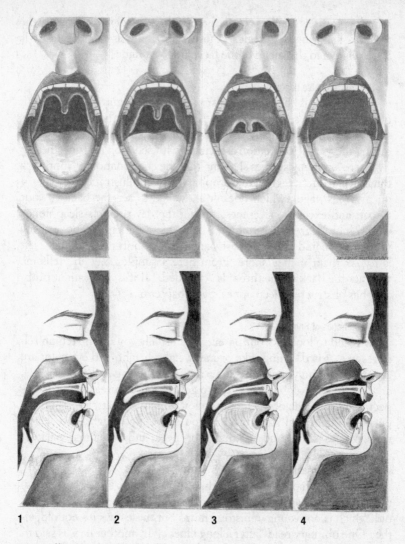

1   2   3   4

Normally you should be able to see the back of your throat, called the posterior (or back) pharyngeal wall. The soft palate ends with the uvula.

When the palate is too long or large or swells from allergies, the trauma of snoring, or another cause, it can produce crowding in the back of the throat and narrow the critical breathing space. If you can see the back of your throat past the uvula, as in position number 1 in the diagram above, that's a good sign. If you can't see the back of your throat, then your palate may be too large or long for the shape of your mouth, position number 4, or there may be swelling owing to the trauma of snoring or allergies. Another possibility is that the palate is large relative to the shape of the face, jaw, or tongue.

Say "Ah" and Live Longer

How useful is the method described above? I may be biased, but offhand I would say "extremely." Anesthesiologists have utilized this simple visual aid for many years to predict if your airway will be safe during the muscle relaxation associated with sedation and anesthesia.

There are many studies showing that the combination of snoring, a thick neck, obesity, crowded oropharynx (i.e., illustration number 4 on previous page), which doesn't allow you to see the back of your throat, and excessive sleepiness during the day predicts sleep apnea with a high degree of certainty. I often see a patient sleeping in my waiting room and if I note obesity and a thick, short neck, all that's left is to ask them if they snore. From here a simple "Say ah" tells me whether the back of the throat is "crowded." If it is, the patient probably has obstructive sleep apnea. See Chapter 6.

The Genetics of Snoring

We tend to look like our parents and usually you can match up relatives in a crowd. Things like overall weight, height, and eye color are examples of family traits. We know now that snoring and apnea as well are often passed along generation to generation. It is reasonable to expect that the inside of the mouth follows inherited patterns, as do the outside craniofacial structures. If you snore, you might have Dad's nose, Mom's jaw, Grandpa's thick short neck, and Grandma's palate!

"After a Long Illness"

We were all saddened to hear that Bob Keeshan, known to generations of fans as Captain Kangaroo, died in early 2004. He was 76 years old, which is not young in historic terms but these days it's not old, either. One obituary read "after a long illness." In another he was said to have been suffering from heart problems since the 1980s.

A number of years prior to his death, when I was new to my practice in sleep medicine, I was watching Captain Kangaroo with my kids. During a great big exaggerated laugh the Captain opened his mouth wide to the camera. The close-up suggested a crowded mouth and large tongue. In retrospect, he may have fit the profile: large neck, crowded throat, and thick gurgly voice.

Such descriptions when taken alone are not specific for sleep apnea. When there is a combination of physical findings such as a crowded throat and a medical history to support the diagnosis, this condition can be suspected with a good degree of certainty.

Step 3: Take a look at your tonsils.

The next step in the self-examination involves looking at how narrow the throat is at the level of the tonsils, right alongside the tip of the uvula or at the end the soft palate. The tonsils are usually hiding out of sight on either side of the tongue in two little cavities called the tonsillar fossae. In adults the tonsils are usually hard to see unless they are swollen by infection or inflammation from disease or allergies. In children, swollen tonsils and adenoids are the most common cause of snoring or obstruction to breathing (see Chapter 12). When the tonsils or tissue near the tonsils enlarge and encroach on the middle of the throat, there is usually significant snoring and cause for concern about further problems such as blockage and apnea. This is seen in frames number 4 and 5 in the diagram below. The position in number 5 is also referred to as the kissing tonsils. The tonsils, crypts, or any tissue in this area may encroach on the airway in this manner, and cause snoring or apnea.

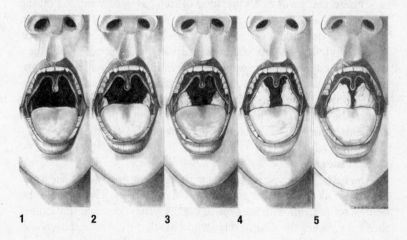

1   2   3   4   5

Step 4: Let it Flow. Let it flow. Let it flow.

Like your throat, the nose and nasopharynx—the narrow passage immediately behind your nostrils—also have both hardware and software. A deviated septum is a hardware problem: The septum, the cartilage that separates the nasal passages from one another, is crooked rather than straight, which disturbs the smooth flow of air through the nose.

The nasopharynx may be the narrowest point along the upper airway and it may need help to keep it open. If you're a typical American male, you watch a fair amount of football on television, and you have surely seen many players wearing little adhesive strips that straddle their noses like butterflies. They do this because it gives them a feeling of unobstructed breathing. In effect it is like widening the opening in the vacuum attachment. Air seems to pass effortlessly through the nose, even during a sprint. The players with the adhesive strips need all the air they can get. And so do you.

To see how nasal dilators work, look in the mirror and sniff hard with your mouth shut. The fleshy outer walls of the nostrils, which are called the **nares,** collapse inward. Now, pinch the nares and pull downward and outward. Try to sniff. What should happen is that by preventing the collapse of the nares, you feel more air moving through at a faster rate to your lungs. Your chest wall doesn't have to work as hard to draw in the air. That greater ease is clearly a boon to a football player—he gains air movement without relying on an open mouth to breathe—difficult to do with a mouthpiece in place.

The sleeper needs that same kind of free passage. Breathing during the various stages of sleep is not uniform. Your body may be at rest, but your mind, depending on your stage of sleep, may be working extra hard. During REM sleep, you may be dreaming about going long for a pass or running away from a monster. Breathing rate and effort change during some stages of sleep. Another principle in airflow physics shows that the faster that air flows through a soft tube the more likely the walls of the tube will collapse in the event of narrowing at the end of the tube. Remember the walls of the airways are very flexible during sleep.

Best Results

The strips work best for people with a narrow nose where the nares look more like a slit rather than the usual oval shape. They can also be helpful for patients with the type of nasal septum deviation that causes the fleshy part of the nose to distort and block the opening. This is discussed in more detail in the treatment section of Chapter 7.

Easy Airflow Test

I use a simple maneuver to test nasal airflow. Begin by blowing your nose so that it is as clear as you can get it. With your mouth closed, block one nostril by placing a finger and pressing on the fleshy outer wall. Now breathe through the unblocked side. Switch sides. If there is a difference in the airflow, you should feel it immediately.

This test only shows that there may be a difference in airflow between the two sides. The nose is a complex structure and there can be many reasons for blockage or partial blockage. An ear, nose, and throat doctor can tell you more about the cause of any differences, such as nasal septum deviation and nasal polyps—growths in the nasal passages—by using a special light called a fiber-optic scope to look from the tip of the nose to the back of the throat. Colds or allergies can produce extra swelling of the tissues and turn partial blockages into very nearly total ones.

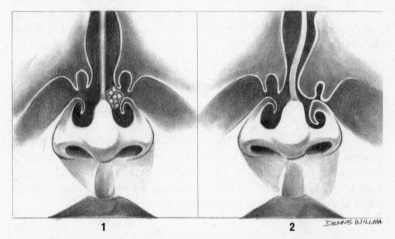

1. On the left is an example of how a grape-sized polyp can block the nasal passage.
2. On the right-hand panel the nasal septum (middle cartilage) is deviated or not straight, narrowing the passsage.

Dry Mouth in the Morning

How does this affect your sleep? Adults normally breathe through their noses as they sleep and if the nose is blocked for any reason, the mouth falls open. The result? Snoring. Have you ever experienced a dry mouth on waking in the morning after a night of a stuffy or blocked nose? This was probably why.

Little-known fact. The sides of the nose alternate breathing duty. They open and close in approximately 90-minute cycles, which seem to coincide with the REM cycle. Think of the problems this can create. If your right side is permanently blocked because of, say, a fixed nasal septum deviation and the left side is on a closed cycle, there will be critical closure on both sides. The result is mouth breathing.

At the sleep center we refer to this by the colorful term "reduced airflow through the nose," which is a prominent item on our list of things that can contribute to snoring and disrupted sleep.

Drip, Drip, Drip

Allergies, which are on the rise in all segments of the population, are a software problem. Not only do the soft tissues of the sinuses swell from inflammation, but the mucous membranes work overtime to exclude pollens and other substances that for most people are totally harmless. The combination of swelling and dripping is a bad one for normal breathing during sleep, because the fluids don't have an opportunity to drain, adding to the likelihood of snoring and disordered breathing during sleep.

The Three-Level Model—Which One Are You?

So far we have discussed how snoring can be traced to the shape of the throat and the state of your upper airway in general. However, there are invisible factors in play as well. Snoring occurs along the air pathways from the tip of the nose to the vocal cords or voice box. As mentioned, we divide these pathways into three parts called the nasopharynx, oropharynx, and hypopharynx. Naturally, some of what takes place in there you can't observe for yourself.

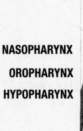
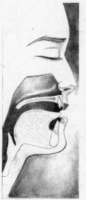

NASOPHARYNX	**LEVEL 1**
OROPHARYNX	**LEVEL 2**
HYPOPHARYNX	**LEVEL 3**

Examples of problems that may contribute to snoring at each of these levels include:

Level 1. Nasal polyps, severe nasal septum deviation, enlargement of the adenoids (spongy tissue between the back of the nose and the throat), small nose, sinusitis (nonallergic inflammation of the sinuses), and allergies

Level 2. Palate enlarged or swollen, uvula enlarged, tonsils enlarged, tongue large, obese neck

Level 3. Bulky back of tongue, small lower jaw (mandible) placed back toward airspace, short or obese neck

Studies have shown that most snoring involves vibration of tissue in some combination of at least two of these three levels, most commonly levels 2 and 3. There are exceptions, however. One example of single-level snoring and associated apnea is the child with enlarged tonsils and adenoids. At the sleep center we often see complete reversal of disordered breathing in children after the tonsils and/or adenoids are taken out. The more common scenario in adults is blockage that occurs when the uvula meets the back of the tongue.

I believe that the role of level-1 problems is underestimated. Obstruction of the nasopharynx lays the groundwork for more advanced levels of breathing dysfunction because the strain on the tissues of the nasopharynx places a burden on other tissues farther back in the airway. Remember the vacuum cleaner: When you obstruct the attachment, the tube farther down the line is prone to collapse as the motor or chest wall strains to pull in more air.

Allergists have a saying: "One airway, one disease," because they see a connection between nasal allergies and asthma. Neglecting nasal allergies increases the chance that allergic inflammation will occur in the rest of the airway. I believe that the same saying also has application for other respiratory issues. In fact, many recent studies stress the importance of "level-1" blockage as a contributing factor in many breathing disorders during sleep.

Level-1 snorers may have no current problems at levels 2 and 3. However, obstruction in the nasopharynx, which is, after all, the first stop for air entry during sleep, reduces the airflow farther back in the airway. Cumulatively, the inflammation and stresses and strains on these initially healthy tissues may change them and make them more prone to blockage later on.

Body Position and Sleep Stage

Snoring is usually worse when we sleep on our backs, because gravity pulls the tongue back against the air passage. This relaxation of the tongue and other soft tissues and muscles in the back of the throat causes partial blockage of the airway, resulting in a loud snore or, in the event of complete blockage, apnea.

During sleep studies, we see the most intense snoring during REM sleep when our subjects are dreaming. This is because their muscles are immobile. When REM sleep is combined with sleeping on their backs, the noise can be pretty intense. (For snorers, sleeping with a partner produces an added hazard—bruising of the ribs. This is not an organic problem. Rather, it results from the continual trauma from the partner's elbow as it smashes into the snorer's rib cage.)

Other factors affecting breathing during sleep are covered in Chapter 6.

In Between Partial Blockage and Total Blockage

Upper airway resistance syndrome is a collection of symptoms, physical findings from a comprehensive doctor's examination, and findings from a sleep laboratory study that are more significant than simple snoring but not as striking as obstructive apnea, which will be described in graphic detail in the next chapter. This condition can be thought of as something between the two in severity yet distinct in several ways. Snoring may be present but is not always. Sleep is disrupted due to narrowing in the upper airway, but without total blockage. The resulting reduced airflow disrupts continuous and restorative sleep with frequent miniarousals that show up on the EEG (electroencephalogram of brain wave activity) during a sleep study but that might not otherwise be detectable. The syndrome may be more common in women and should be considered when the cause of excessive daytime sleepiness is not clear.

When snoring is very severe but not associated with definite obstruction or apnea, and when there is a personal history of hypertension and cardiovascular disease, some sleep specialists call it *Heavy Snorer's Disease*. There is more and more evidence to support the notion that severe snoring damages surrounding structures. It also worsens with obesity. Since obesity is also a risk factor for other bad conditions such as hypertension, diabetes, and high cholesterol, there may be some overlap of associated disease. Heavy snoring may be the calling card. However, since not every person who snores loudly has these other medical problems, more study is obviously needed to identify other indicators to make it easier to distinguish heavy snoring from Heavy Snorer's Disease. Research in the area is currently focusing on genetic risk factors or unique combinations of anatomy and body chemistry that might turn up in laboratory tests.

Regardless of whether you have Heavy Snorer's Disease or are merely a heavy snorer, the problem should be treated.

Snoring may be a sign of a serious medical problem. If you have concerns after reading this chapter, talk to your doctor, who may refer you to an ear, nose, and throat (ENT) specialist. The information obtained from an ENT examination is combined with the rest of your history and examination to arrive at a likely diagnosis. Bottom line: I believe that any sound you emit regularly from your mouth or nose during sleep is not a normal part of restful sleep. Snoring is no exception.

6

SLEEP APNEA—WHEN BREATHING STOPS

TAKE THE SLEEP APNEA TEST

	Yes	No

1. Do you snore regularly?
2. Do you stop breathing or gasp during sleep?
3. Do you have high blood pressure?
4. Are you overweight with a 16½-inch or larger collar size?

If you answered yes to all four questions, the chances are good that you have obstructive sleep apnea, and believe me, this is not a test where you want a high score. Other predisposing factors include gender—males have a higher rate of apnea than females by a two-to-one margin—and age, with people ages 40 to 75 particularly vulnerable.

Need more evidence? Answer the following:

5. Do you awaken feeling tired or unrefreshed?
6. Do you wake up with a headache or a dry mouth?
7. Do you feel tired enough to nap during the day?
8. Do you have episodes of impotence?
9. Are you aware of changes in your personality?

If you have these symptoms, along with a high score on questions one through four, the chances that you have sleep apnea increase.

Dial 911

As Mrs. Smith remembered it, this is how the emergency call went:

"Send an ambulance! My husband is choking! He's holding his throat!"

"Ma'am, slow down. Do you know the Heimlich maneuver?"

"He didn't eat anything. It's 3 A.M., for God's sake. He's asleep and he's choking."

Fortunately for Mr. Smith, his wife managed to rouse him from his sleep. But, of course, the health crisis didn't end when he woke up. Mr. Smith was suffering from the most extreme form of obstructive sleep apnea. He choked like this many times a night. Picture the poster you see in every restaurant directing you to do the Heimlich maneuver—the victim's hands are clutching his throat. Imagine being in that state of panic routinely. Think of the shock to your system. That's what is happening to you at night if you have sleep apnea, and you aren't even aware of it.

What does it take to produce that kind of panic? Maybe you have watched your child bite off too much hot dog and have it get stuck on the way down. Maybe someone you know has had too much to drink, cut off a piece of steak half the size of a pack of cigarettes, and greedily tried to swallow it before chewing thoroughly. Their whole demeanor changes. Their eyes bulge in panic. They wave their hands to get the attention of their fellow diners and start to gesture wildly at their throats. They might be able to grunt, but they can't say anything because no air can pass through their vocal cords.

The realization of what is happening to them is terrible. Their whole life doesn't pass before their eyes, at least not right away. There's still enough time before they lose consciousness to do something about it, if they can get their companions to do the right thing—but that's a big if and the uncertainty is excruciating.

In the case of sleep apnea, your upper airway has already been narrowed by overweight, allergies, or chronic inflammation of the tissues, and all it takes is your tongue or uvula falling across the remaining space to cause you to choke. Then your body goes into panic mode, only you aren't awake to experience that panic. Maybe if you were, you might have done something about it a long time ago.

The symptoms of sleep apnea are so ugly to witness that even unschooled observers recognize that there is something wrong. Published studies from our sleep center and others indicate that if your bed partner is sufficiently alarmed to urge you to go to the doctor by what she (for it is usually "she"—most patients with undiagnosed sleep apnea are men) sees, there is a very good chance that you have the condition.

Enough to Spoil Your Dinner

The Heimlich maneuver was invented in the mid-1970s. What happened to people who were choking on their food at restaurants before that? If they were lucky, there was a doctor in the house who could perform an emergency tracheotomy with a steak knife. The good samaritan doctor would open a hole in the neck and then one in the windpipe so the victim could breathe. A tracheotomy is one of the oldest recorded surgical procedures and is even depicted in Egyptian hieroglyphics.

In a hospital, under controlled conditions, a plastic tube is also inserted, in order to provide a more stable opening, a procedure called tracheostomy. In cases where there is no obstruction, the preferred procedure is oral-tracheal intubation, in which a long plastic tube is inserted through the mouth and pushed past the windpipe and vocal cords in order to help get air and/or oxygen into the lungs. In fact, as you will read, when undiagnosed sleep apnea is confused with heart attacks, congestive heart failure, or lung disease—as it often is in emergency rooms—intubation plays a big part in treatment.

Your Body to the Rescue

Sleep apnea activates your sympathetic nervous system. Have you ever heard those stories about people gaining enough strength in an emergency to lift a car off an accident victim? That's the sympathetic nervous system in action. Have you ever run for a bus much farther and faster than you imagined you could? That, too, is the sympathetic nervous system. (It's only after you have boarded the bus and paid your fare that you feel like you might have a heart attack.)

Not every activation of the sympathetic nervous system is helpful. Have you ever had a screaming match with someone, a truly uncontrollable fit of rage? Again, that is your sympathetic nervous system. It takes a while to recover from, doesn't it? You feel worn out, maybe guilty for losing control, and often disconcerted by the force of your reaction.

All of these examples are concerned with a vital "fight-or-flight" response that was created to be used sparingly. Remember the phrase "survival of the fittest"? This was part of it. Our ancestors did not always occupy modern man's privileged spot at the top of the food chain, and they needed this response to help protect themselves from predators. This nervous system override of mind and body is discussed in detail in Chapter 10 on insomnia.

Think of your body as a city. Normally, it functions pretty well. The schools are open five days a week during the school year. The sanitation trucks collect garbage. The police and the fire departments do their jobs of keeping you and your homes safe. Taxes and services more or less stay in balance. Generally everyone lives a quiet life.

Suddenly, there is an epidemic of arson accompanied by a crime wave. The police departments and fire departments have to be on continual alert, responding to real emergencies as well as doing their usual jobs. The taxpayers have to pay them lots of overtime. The police and firefighters are getting injured and suffering from exhaustion at abnormally high rates. Their vehicles race from one incident to another, burning lots of gasoline and requiring extra maintenance. The money and resources needed for all these additional expenses are siphoned from school budgets and street repair and garbage collection funds. In the meantime, our children go uneducated, our streets fill with potholes, and our towns and cities get shabbier.

Well, obstructive sleep apnea is this kind of municipal emergency in the body hundreds of times a night. After a while, your body is like that city—run-down and falling apart.

Red Alert

One of the first systems to show the stress of obstructed breathing is the respiratory system, which experiences "negative intrathoracic pressure." In plain English, this means your chest is trying to pull air through a hose—the pharynx—that is critically narrowed or completely blocked. This leads in turn to the flight-or-fight response discussed above. The surge from the sympathetic nervous system, complete with the adrenaline-like jolts, causes fluctuations in heart rate and "increased vascular resistance," which is a well-known blood vessel response in most types of high blood pressure. Too much blood is trying to go through too narrow a pipeline. Many current studies suggest that in time this temporary heart and blood vessel response turns into chronic hypertension and related vascular disease, at which point your GP or cardiologist will appropriately start to treat it with medication.

Less obvious is what is happening to the blood pressure at night as your body undergoes repeated episodes of silent suffocation. Sleep apnea patients often have blood-oxygen levels as low as 80 percent. This means your vital tissues and organs aren't getting the oxygen they need. Readings of 90 percent or less are enough to send an otherwise healthy person to the emergency room.

The exchange of oxygen for carbon dioxide is also impaired. Carbon dioxide is a by-product of breathing—the exhaust from your body after the red blood cells have delivered fresh oxygen to the cells. Do you remember what happened in the movie *Beverly Hills Cop* when Eddie Murphy put bananas in the tailpipe of the unmarked police car being driven by detectives assigned to keep track of his movements? The car stalled. Fortunately, in the case of obstructive sleep apnea, the engine restarts, just in time, after every respiratory stall. But what a stress to the body! No wonder patients with untreated apnea are tired the next day. Although you wake up before you suffocate, those repeated miniarousals interrupt your restorative sleep. Left untreated, they are measurably terrible for you and your quality of life in the long run. These episodes not only deprive your vital tissues and organs of the chance to recover from the wear and tear of everyday life during sleep, as you are supposed to, but they age you mentally.

We compute the severity of apnea by the apnea index, which is the total number of apnea episodes during sleep divided by the total number of hours of sleep, a relative measure of apnea severity. An apnea index of five or more defines the presence of obstructive sleep apnea.

Research has shown that when you have 15 apnea episodes per hour of sleep, a moderate number, the effect on your performance on neuropsychological tests is the equivalent of adding five years to your age. Consider, then, that some people experience these apnea episodes 50–100 times *an hour*.

Last Gasp, 400 Times a Night

We call your body's violent, ultimate defense the last gasp, or last-gasp resuscitation. When your uvula and/or tongue is blocking your windpipe like a cork in a bottle, a neurochemical process is triggered. Oxygen and carbon dioxide levels change in your blood since the normal rhythmic movement of air in and out of your body is interrupted. Fresh oxygen can't be delivered. Your body sends the alarm "I'm going to die if I don't get some air!" That message goes to the brain, which swings into action, giving your diaphragm a neurochemical jolt. A sudden violent contraction wakes the muscles in the entire breathing circuit and a loud explosive gasp unplugs the obstruction, allowing air to enter the lungs. Just in time!

Your brain is commanding your body to do the Heimlich maneuver 400 times a night, only instead of a piece of steak, it is dislodging a part of your body. Not a pretty picture. And not good for you.

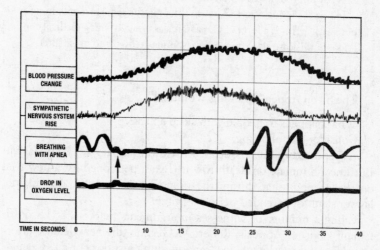

In this graphic representation breathing stops at the first arrow. The nervous system reacts to the stress causing a rise in blood pressure while blood oxygen levels fall in response to the apnea.

Flatline to frantic: As you can see on the left of the chart on the previous page, the patient has stopped breathing. Ten seconds later, the oxygen level has fallen. It actually falls slowly because thankfully we all have some reserve stores in our tissues and blood. With severe and repeated apnea, however, or in those with lung or heart disease, these reserves are depleted and after 10 to 20 seconds there is a serious drop in oxygen picked up by the oxygen sensor on the finger or earlobe during the sleep study. The nervous system is very sensitive to signals of suffocation, a real stress, and as a protective mechanism it swings into action. The result is depicted in the top two lines with a response from the nervous system and blood pressure that reflects the resuscitative gasp that brings in vital oxygen. This explosion is a lifesaving event, but at what cost to your body?

Gratuitous Violence

W. S. came to me with severe sleep apnea. His last-gasp resuscitation was so violent that during his sleep apnea episodes he thrashed about and broke three televisions and assorted other furniture over a period of several months. This was not a guy you would want to mess with. He's a security officer.

"What did you do?" I asked his wife. "This could be dangerous."

"I know," she answered. "I haven't slept in the same bed with him for four years." This is a form of parasomnia associated with a medical condition, in this case sleep apnea. Parasomnia is discussed in Chapter 9.

The Sleep Apnea "Walking Wounded"

What happens to people with sleep apnea?

Consider the following:

As reported by the Associated Press on January 22, 2001, Calvin Burdine, an inmate on death row in Texas, petitioned for a new trial on the grounds that during the original trial in 1984, the original lawyer slept for extended periods of time.

Citing a number of witnesses in arguments before the U.S. Fifth Circuit Court of Appeals, Robert McGlasson, the new defense attorney claimed that "the *late* Joe Cannon didn't just doze or daydream—he was unconscious . . . An unconscious lawyer can't object, can't rebut an argument and can't effectively cross-examine a witness" (emphasis added).

Burdine had come within moments of execution in 1987 before a reprieve was granted.

Cannon's excuse, according to other press accounts, was that he was "not asleep, but closed his eyes to concentrate."

Now, I was not Mr. Cannon's doctor, so I don't know what his diagnosis was. He is dead, and as of this writing I haven't been able to find an obituary, so I don't know what killed him. However, based on the testimony of those who observed him in the courtroom, I would say that at the time of the trial, in all likelihood he had a sleep-wake disorder or at least one of the disorders associated with excessive daytime sleepiness (see Chapter 4). When an unjust, or just, courtroom verdict hangs in the balance, and the death penalty is on the table, all eyes should be wide open.

The uncontrollable urge to doze during conversation and then denying that you were sleepy are classic signs. We use them in our clinic to help zero in on a diagnosis. I believe that variations on Mr. Cannon's story are repeated millions of times a day, although they don't always make the headlines. Drivers fall asleep at the wheel, and property is damaged and people are injured. Dozing factory workers make mistakes, and the quality of the things they make is compromised—think about that when your new car makes an annoying rattle or you need to have it repaired after only 10,000 miles. Even doctors have sleep apnea. It's just a matter of time before sleep apnea will show up on a TV program like *ER,* just as it did on an episode of *The Sopranos.*

Even if there is no immediate danger to others, these people are dying a slow death, suffering needless misery, and inflicting distress on their families, colleagues, and friends.

The career of a person with untreated severe sleep apnea follows a predictable pattern—a gradual decline in attention span and productivity, onset of "unrelated" medical conditions, and eventually disability.

Sleep Apnea and the NFL Point Spread

According to a 2002 study by Sleep Tech Consulting Group, in conjunction with ResMed Inc., of more than 300 players from eight teams, 14 percent of National Football League players have sleep apnea, a figure that rises to 34 percent among NFL linemen. Think about that the next time you bet on the Super Bowl. Which team has the higher number of apnea sufferers? You'll never know at the opening kickoff, but if the defensive line starts to run out of steam in the second half, you might get some idea. Is someone taking longer to recover from an injury than originally projected? It could be that he's not giving his body a chance to get better by getting the requisite amount of restorative sleep.

Like the rest of us, those muscular giants need a good night's sleep. They have been superbly conditioned in most respects. NFL trainers have diet and exercise regimens down to a science. But as they have belatedly recognized, sleep is just as important to player conditioning as the other factors. Dr. Allan M. Levy, team physician for the New York Giants, says, "Sleep is the next logical final performance frontier."

If the statistics are disturbing for football players, they are even worse for sumo wrestlers. In its March 12, 2003 edition, *Japan Times Today* reported a study showing that half the sumo wrestlers at a Tokyo stable had been found to suffer from sleep disordered breathing, and linked the condition to poor performance in the ring. The study was initiated by Naohito Suzuki, a doctor of allergy and respiratory disease at Douai Memorial Hospital in Tokyo's Sumida Ward, after an incident in which a Shinkansen bullet-train driver on the JR Sanyo Line nodded off at the controls.

The study, which measured the wrestlers' blood-oxygen saturation while they slept, showed that 11 out of 23 had some degree of sleep-disordered breathing, and that six of these had a serious problem, probably apnea.

The problem showed up in their winning percentages. Those suffering from the disorder won an average of 41 percent of their matches, while their healthier peers won an average of 50 percent of theirs.

However, bad as the prognosis is for sumo wrestlers, who are obviously obese although fantastically dexterous and energetic, the most disturbing part of this news item is the mention of the train driver. Professional athletes in the United States, Japan, and everywhere else will probably receive treatment for their sleep apnea. It's the train drivers of the world we must really worry about, as well as ferry pilots, oil tanker captains, pilots, air traffic controllers, soccer moms and dads— the list is very long.

Sleep Apnea and Overweight

Every week we seem to be assaulted with new evidence that Americans of all ages are gaining weight. This puts us at higher risk of sleep apnea.

Every year the National Sleep Foundation awards what it calls "Pickwick Postdoctoral Sleep Research Fellowships." The fellowships are named after a boy in Charles Dickens's *The Pickwick Papers* named Joe, who was badly overweight and tended to fall asleep essentially whenever he sat down.

In the decades after the publication of *The Pickwick Papers,* doctors would refer to this character when they encountered an obese person with this tendency toward pathological sleepiness. The term *Pickwickian syndrome* was commonly applied to such a case, and those with sleep apnea were noted to have a Pickwickian build. We now apply it to a very specific group of patients with chronic respiratory failure, heart failure, and many symptoms similar to those of patients with sleep apnea.

The link is not necessarily between fat and apnea. For example, football players are conditioned for muscle mass with low body fat. A good deal of that bulk ends up around their neck and chest wall. The effect on their breathing appears to be the same as in obese patients with obstructive sleep apnea due to fatty tissue in the same areas.

I recently saw a weightlifter who at, six feet three inches, 335 pounds, was very fit. He also had severe obstructive sleep apnea. All that hard-earned muscle was no doubt deprived of normal oxygen levels as he slept. Muscle repair and growth occurs during sleep and a proper balance of nutrients, oxygen, and natural hormones (he did not take supplements) is needed to get the best results. He was very willing to use CPAP, especially when I suggested that the therapy may help him bench-press his goal of 703 pounds in preparation for upcoming competition. "I want the gold" he said.

Apnea is linked to anatomical features other than weight. Many "nonobese" people suffer from apnea due to the shape of the bones and tissues in their faces and necks. Some studies for example suggest that Mexicans and certain Asians particularly are prone to apnea without being conspicuously overweight.

Even marginal weight gain to levels not considered otherwise harmful can make a crucial difference. Whether the new pounds come from muscle or flab, the linkage is clear. Research indicates that a mere 10 percent weight gain correlates with a six-times-greater risk of sleep apnea.

World News Roundup: Apnea Links to High Blood Pressure, Heart Disease, and Other Serious Trouble

You may recall that earlier in this book I stated that problems that are sleep-related are often treated separately, and expensively, without a careful screening for nighttime risk factors. Among the conditions that reflect the complexity of the 24-hour day are three of the most common that doctors in general medical practice encounter—high blood pressure, heart disease, and diabetes. The links between sleep apnea and these conditions are proven, and I have no doubt that in time many other medical problems will be similarly tied to sleep disorders.

APNEA AND CARDIOVASCULAR DISEASE

Dateline Gothenburg, Sweden:

A team of Swedish scientists studied middle-aged men, some with sleep apnea and some without, over a period of seven years. At the beginning of the study, none of the subjects suffered from a list of conditions such as hypertension or other cardiovascular disease, pulmonary disease, diabetes, or alcoholism. After accounting for such factors as body mass, smoking, blood pressure, and age, those with untreated sleep apnea eventually exhibited some form of cardiovascular disease at a rate nearly six times (22 of 60 or 37.7 percent) the rate of those treated for sleep apnea (8 of 122 or 6.7 percent). Moreover, out of 15 subjects who were efficiently treated for apnea, only one experienced cardiovascular disease, compared with 21 out of 37 for those who were inadequately treated.

APNEA AND HIGH BLOOD PRESSURE

Dateline Madison, Wisconsin:

University of Wisconsin scientists analyzed data on patients with sleep-disordered breathing, including data on blood pressure level, and such factors as smoking and alcohol consumption. After four years, 709 of them were retested and after eight years 184 were tested again. The study showed that the more apnea events these people suffered per hour of sleep, the more likely they were to have high blood pressure.

This study shows that like smoking, obesity, and other well-known contributing factors, sleep apnea by itself can contribute to high blood pressure.

APNEA AND ARRHYTHMIA

Dateline Dublin, Ireland:

Most people without heart disease have fairly regular heartbeats between midnight and 6 A.M. However, for those with sleep apnea, all those hormonal jolts keep their hearts from relaxing the way they should. Researchers in Ireland studied 8 subjects from a group of 17 sleep apnea patients (45 percent) who had nighttime heart arrhythmia—irregular heartbeats—between 11 P.M. and 7 A.M. The particular problems they experienced included pauses of 2 to 10 seconds, premature ventricular contractions, and second-degree atrioventricular block, which is a short circuit and blockage of the electrical signal in the heart. In effect, the heart does not beat when it should. More recent studies done in several centers showed the association of atrial fibrillation, another fairly common heart arrhythmia, with untreated sleep apnea.

In most cases the arrhythmias improved after their apnea was treated with CPAP (continuous positive air pressure). In the Dublin study, the one patient who did not respond favorably had other problems, and eventually needed heart valve replacement surgery.

Dateline Marburg, Germany:

If apnea itself is a risk factor for hypertension, as the above-mentioned study shows, then treatment ought to reduce the incidence of the "silent killer," as high blood pressure is known, and recently German researchers have shown that it does.

Patients who received therapeutic CPAP treatment experienced improvement in their blood pressure both at night and during the day. The drop in mean blood pressure of 10mm Hg registered during the study— from 140/90 to 130/80, for example—would probably reduce the risk of coronary artery disease by 37 percent and stroke risk by 56 percent.

Not too shabby.

APNEA AND ENLARGED HEART

Dateline Salt Lake City:

Researchers have found that for people with sleep apnea, the left side of the heart often becomes enlarged. Fortunately, apnea treatment can reverse the process.

A team led by Dr. Tom V. Cloward at Latter-Day Saints (LDS) Hospital's Intermountain Sleep Disorders Center in Salt Lake City, Utah, used echocardiography to measure the hearts of 25 patients with severe obstructive sleep apnea before and after they were treated.

Twenty-three of the 25 subjects showed abnormalities in the structure of their hearts, and 22 of those had left-sided enlargement. Thirteen of the patients had both high blood pressure and enlarged hearts.

Twenty of the patients who complied with CPAP therapy showed significant improvement in the size of their hearts, the team reports. Those who were unable to persist with treatment showed no such benefit or significant change.

Dateline France:

French researchers, after observing that men with sleep apnea also showed early signs of diabetes, tested the blood of 700 men suspected of having sleep apnea after a "meal" of glucose.

They found that approximately half showed signs of a diabetes-related metabolic disorder.

Nearly one in three of those with confirmed apnea could actually be classified as diabetic, two-fifths of whom were previously undiagnosed.

Moreover, as one of the researchers said, "the degree of insulin resistance correlated with the severity of the sleep apnea." Furthermore, even snorers without apnea have trouble metabolizing sugar. As discussed in Chapter 5 not all people who snore have apnea; however, snoring has its own set of health concerns.

Researchers theorize that apnea alters stress hormones and oxygen utilization in a way that interferes with insulin's job of getting sugar into cells.

ATTENTION-DEFICIT/HYPERACTIVITY DISORDER

Dateline Augusta, Georgia:

While childhood attention-deficit/hyperactivity disorder (ADHD) has suffered from no deficit of parental and teacher attention (and I will have a lot more to say about it later in this book), its symptoms persist well past childhood and so do treatments, usually involving a stimulant such as Ritalin. As sleep doctors have long known, the symptoms of ADHD can be remarkably similar to those of sleep apnea.

Successful treatment of three men, ages 19, 23, and 44 with persistent ADHD at a Georgia sleep center indicates that sleep medicine is a very exciting new frontier for this troubling epidemic among children and adults alike.

All three men were overweight and all three had been treated for symptoms that included daytime sleepiness and short attention spans. All had airway blockages, and their sleep studies showed moderate to severe sleep apnea and inadequate oxygen saturation. Two of them were treated with CPAP machines, while the third chose weight loss and medical treatment for his nasal congestion.

In each case, their daytime symptoms improved and all three were weaned from their dependence on stimulants. The overlap of symptoms for ADHD and sleep apnea has obvious treatment implications and as such is an area of ongoing and much needed research.

Dateline Quebec, Canada:

Professor Yves Lacasse and his colleagues at the Center for Pneumology at Laval University, Quebec, utilized a quality-of-life scale developed for patients with asthma or chronic bronchitis to assess middle-aged patients suffering from sleep apnea.

More than two-thirds reported feeling impatient, 59 percent felt anxious, and 53 percent felt depressed.

Nearly 80 percent experienced excessive daytime sleepiness, which affected their emotional well-being. Professor Lacasse says: "It was a surprise for us to find such a large number of depressed patients in our group. . . . Patients are always tired, they have problems at work, problems with their spouse, they don't go out because they know that they will fall asleep, they are even reluctant to go out with friends."

In some cases depression is a self-reinforcing condition whatever the impetus, whether it is sleep deprivation or a traumatic event. The traumatic events can't be undone, but sleep apnea can.

Spotting Sleep Apnea

This is an exciting time to be involved in sleep medicine because once patients get the message, they become a great source of new information. They also become adept at recognizing the daytime symptoms of apnea among family, friends, and colleagues, and urging them to seek an evaluation.

They are good at this because the signs are really pretty easy to recognize once you know what to look for, and once they "get religion" as the result of feeling so much better after treatment, these patients become willing evangelists.

When Nature Calls

Terence, a banker, used to wake up repeatedly at night to urinate. He attributed this to the normal plumbing indignities that arrive with middle-age and told himself, one of these days I must go to a urologist. Of more immediate concern—to his wife—was the noise and sight of Terence snorting and choking in his sleep. Finally he went to a doctor who diagnosed apnea and put him on a CPAP machine. Not only did he begin sleeping through the night without the symptoms of apnea, he stopped getting up to go to the bathroom.

Curious about the coincidence, he asked his doctor about whether there was a connection. There was.

During an episode of apnea—up to 400 times a night—your body sends a distress signal telling it to expel blocked tissue from the airway and start breathing again.

At that point, your heart chambers and blood vessels in your chest have been stressed and there is a reflexive signal to change blood pressure (refer to the diagram on page 87). After repeated signals over time the body responds with a protective chemical reflex and attempts to lower the blood pressure. One of the ways to accomplish this is by getting rid of sodium and water, and the best way to do that is to urinate. So your heart secretes something called naturetic hormone, which helps fill your bladder and eventually wakes you to urinate.

There's another explanation, a kind of a folk tale, which says that when your sleep is inadequate, your kidneys continue to function as if you were awake. Not true. You form more urine at night as a result of sleep apnea than you do during normal waking hours.

Cool Sleep Fact—*Native American Alarm Clock*

Indian warriors derived part of their advantage from surprising their enemies, and the way they generally achieved it was to attack before their foes could attack them. Before they went to sleep on the eve of a battle, they would drink extra water. As a consequence, their own urges would awaken them before dawn.

Apnea and Your Body Clock

Your body operates on a schedule. As explained earlier, this is called circadian rhythm. During the hours from 2 A.M. through 10 A.M., for example, when your body tends to be at its thirstiest because you haven't been drinking fluids, your blood platelets are sticky and your blood is thicker than usual. Not coincidentally, these are also the peak hours for heart attacks.

Most organs and systems in your body are influenced by circadian rhythms, and are thrown out of kilter by the effects of interrupted breathing.

For example, at night, the bronchi—small airways in the lungs—are narrowed from their daytime circumference. They are dilated only enough to accommodate the relatively minimal needs of a resting body. However, because they are minimally dilated, they are also more sensitive to bronchoconstriction. This is an additional problem for asthmatics who are very sensitive to the allergens that abound in beds because of the large numbers of dust mites that inhabit them, feeding on dead skin.

When these allergens provoke a typical allergic reaction in the already constricted bronchi, the result is a disproportionate incidence of asthma compared with the rest of the day. The problem is even more serious for asthmatics who also have sleep apnea. Asthma is a condition that brings many threads of the 24-hour story of human health together and underscores the necessity of a multidisciplinary approach to treatment.

Asthma and allergies have a genetic component, as sleep apnea often does. This genetic condition is triggered by environmental factors—dust and other allergens—and they collide with circadian and immunologic changes in the airways during sleep. The result can be catastrophic.

Sleep Apnea and Gastroesophageal Reflux Disorder (GERD)

Questions 14–18 on the test in Chapter 1 dealt with gastroesophageal reflux disorder, which results from stomach acid backing up into the throat during the night. The significance of these questions lies in the fact that a very high percentage of those with GERD also have sleep apnea. When acid backs up into the throat, it irritates and inflames the tissues that are involved in attacks of sleep apnea. ENT doctors who treat these people can see the corrosive effects of acid reflux on these tissues.

As with many issues in sleep medicine, there's some question about whether apnea triggers reflux, or the other way around. Some researchers believe that apnea leads to changes in airway pressure, causing reflux to occur. Other researchers think that the reflux of acids causes spasms of the tissues around the vocal cords and subsequently triggers apnea.

In any case, treatment for sleep apnea, notably CPAP, has also been shown to help reduce symptoms of GERD. Likewise, antacids that help with GERD may have beneficial effects on sleep apnea.

Heart Attack or Obstructive Sleep Apnea?

I do rounds every day with hospital residents and interns. We will arrive at an ICU bed where a patient is fully sedated, surrounded by the monitoring systems, and on a mechanical ventilator. I will present these young doctors with a chart from the initial work-up and ask them for diagnosis.

Blood pressure erratic. Blood oxygen—too low. Sodium imbalance. Water retention excessive. Pulse erratic.

When they see the above symptoms, generally they will diagnose coronary artery disease, myocardial disease, pump damage, congestive heart failure, pulmonary edema, or other catastrophic conditions. And usually they are right.

Five or six times a year, however, they see a different cause for this heart and lung failure. What they are really seeing is *untreated* obstructive sleep apnea, which has mimicked the symptoms of these other conditions.

In each case, the patient has been intubated—that is, a breathing tube has been placed directly in the airway past the obstruction that over months or years got them into trouble in the first place. Within two to three days, the apnea patients are fully recovered. They typically pass six to seven gallons of water. Their lungs clear of fluid and their blood gasses return to normal. They are fully alert. In fact, when off the ventilator and able to talk one of the first things they say is that they feel better than they have in years.

The Heart-Apnea Connection

Of course, when those patients come out of the ICU "feeling better than ever," their problems are not over. They still need treatment for the condition. Their hearts have adjusted to working under adverse conditions every night. Severe apnea of this type is akin to "part-time heart failure," with heart, lungs, and brain straining every night to get both the normal amounts of blood and oxygen they need and supply them to other vital tissues. Every morning these people wake up groggy, grouchy, and often with a headache.

It takes an hour or more to get out of this state of temporary heart failure and, if they are lucky, ready to start their day. As with anything that forces the heart to strain hard—fat in your coronary arteries, high blood pressure, chronic lung disease—apnea puts you in danger of bigger problems down the road. Apnea puts the chambers of the heart under stress, every night, or one third of every 24 hours. In severe cases, especially those where the heart is already damaged, damage is compounded by apnea episodes. In one study of patients with apnea, the walls of the heart were shown on echocardiograms to be thicker than they should be as a result of the straining at night. These changes reversed after CPAP treatment.

It's a vicious cycle. A combination of any conditions like high blood pressure, diabetes, high cholesterol, smoking, and the rest of the murderers' row of modern ailments dramatically increases risk of cardiovascular disease over a long period of time.

The heart-sleep connection, therefore, is a key area of sleep research at our center. We studied 136 patients with sleep apnea and found that the electrocardiogram (ECG) revealed a "footprint" called a "Q-T interval change" in many patients with sleep apnea. The Q-T interval is measured on the ECG in seconds and reflects the time it takes for the heart to get ready for the next heartbeat. It is very important that this electrical activity be absolutely regular. Changes in this recovery time have been found to contribute to heart dysfunction and dangerous and sometimes deadly arrhythmias in other well-studied heart disease populations such as heart attack patients. We are looking at the footprints to explain similar complications in patients with sleep apnea. Our research shows a high incidence of abnormalities unexplained by any other well-known associations or factors such as use of medication or damage to the heart itself. There is ample evidence to show that apnea is changing the electrical activity in your heart, putting you at risk for long-term complications.

You Don't Know What a Good Night's Sleep Is

Many apnea patients don't really know what "normal" is like—to feel alert, energetic, and headache-free. This absence of "normality" takes its toll on their well-being in both obvious and subtle ways. Yet, they are slow to seek treatment, and once they do seek help, they are often reluctant to make the changes they need to make.

In a way, patients who arrive in the ICU are fortunate because they are urgently resuscitated and intubated. The close call and the relief they experience makes them feel truly reborn when they wake up.

They are learning the hard way how it feels to breathe without an obstruction, but they are learning it, and they love it.

Those who find their way to a sleep center by way of the front door instead of via the emergency room have to make some choices, and they are often reluctant to do so. A reporter for *The New York Times* who wrote about his experience at a sleep center and about trying CPAP declined to continue using the machine. This is too bad. It takes a bit of getting used to—sleeping with an air compressor next to your bed which delivers air into your body through a mask that fits over the nose and mouth. In the TV show *The Sopranos,* Uncle Junior is fitted with a CPAP machine, and observes that he looks like a fighter pilot, although in somewhat more colorful language. I say, if it's good enough for the Sopranos, it should be good enough for the *Times.*

Regardless, I have a feeling that some day if he wants to be insured, the writer will have to agree to treatment. The cost of untreated apnea, measured in additional treatment of heart disease, diabetes, depression, and so on, is roughly double the cost for those who are treated. But while the financial costs can be calculated by insurance companies and government statisticians, the big picture ignores the cost to the lives of individuals, families, coworkers, and many others of untreated apnea.

I don't blame people for their reluctance to comply with treatment. They are wedded to their habits and their habits are often based on the compromises we all make in a busy, complicated world. A couple of meals at McDonald's every week may save a person time and money over healthier alternatives, but if the price he pays is an extra half-inch in his shirt collar size, he pays for it every night and every day.

Fortunately, there's a way around that oversized collar that doesn't necessarily involve losing weight—although that would be advisable in cases where weight gain is contributing to apnea—in the form of the CPAP, which will be discussed in greater detail in Chapter 7.

I cut right to the chase with apnea patients. I tell them, in effect, "You don't know what a good night's sleep is." They are so accustomed to sleeping badly that they have nothing to compare it with, sort of like a smoker who doesn't know what food really tastes like or how good fresh air smells. Feeling lousy during the day is "normal" to people with apnea.

I ask them to try CPAP to establish a baseline for treatment. To many of these people the experience is a revelation because in the very short term, the payoffs are dramatic. They learn how it feels to awake refreshed and then spend the rest of the day free of the headaches, dozing, and depression that they are accustomed to. This experience alone is enough to put many patients on the road to recovery. Since compliance with the CPAP is so essential to recovery we invite all patients who have initial problems with the treatments back to the center for further review. Still, CPAP is not the only treatment as I will explain in the next chapter, and it may in fact only be required in the short term; with weight loss and other treatment of the airway, some patients may be able to avoid permanent CPAP use.

Mario the Shoe Salesman

Every morning in the summer on my way to work I would pass Mario's shoe store. He was often asleep in a chair on the sidewalk next to his "final sale" display. Final sale indeed. Mario was a poster child for sleep apnea—overweight, short, thick neck, swollen legs revealed by his Bermuda shorts, and above all the inability to stay *awake*.

One day I got a call to see Mario in the hospital to evaluate him for respiratory failure. Why was I not surprised?

After liberating him from the ventilator and about twenty pounds of water, I treated his apnea with a CPAP machine. The result was dramatic. He couldn't remember when he had last slept so peacefully.

I was well rewarded for my efforts—I got a bear hug during my morning rounds, along with a promise for "any shoe in the store."

Sleep to Save Your Sex Life

The expression "time for bed" has two common meanings, only one of which has to do with sleeping. Snoring is an impediment to both.

Part of the problem is sensory. In most relationships, at least occasionally one partner or the other will awaken a sleeping partner with some loving gestures and coax them into romantic activity.

This is unlikely to happen when the sleeping partner sounds like faulty plumbing. For one thing, the odds of amorous activity being initiated spontaneously are slim, because in many cases the partner is already occupying a separate bedroom. A study of 4,900 patients by the Center for Corrective Jaw Surgery in Philadelphia shows that this is the case with 80 percent of couples in which one is a serious snorer.

For another, snoring can make either partner too tired or too irritable for nature to take its course. For men, it can interfere with the ability to get an erection. According to Dr. Max Hirshkowitz of the Baylor

College of Medicine, who has conducted two relevant studies, "We found that people with severe sleep apnea have, on average, lower testosterone." But supplementing their natural levels of testosterone produces a kind of hormonal double jeopardy—additional testosterone increases the severity of their sleep apnea.

In a study conducted at the National Naval Medical Center in Bethesda, Maryland, 29 men and 3 women who were being newly treated with CPAP machines were asked to rate their sex lives before and after treatment.

What did they find?

Surprise, surprise.

After treatment both their sex drive and the quality of their orgasms improved. Janet Myers, who led the research team, said: "In men, sexual dysfunction may be related to suppression of reproductive or hormonal functioning." She also said that diminished blood oxygen levels could hinder erection. (Engorgement in erectile tissue is a factor in sexual performance and pleasure for both men and women.)

Sleeping Next to a Machine

How long does it take to get used to sleeping next to a person who needs a machine to breathe properly? No time at all, according to W. C., a postal worker who has been using a CPAP machine for more than two years.

"My wife could sleep through anything and was initially unaware of the problem." As is true of many patients with sleep disorders, W. C. was also oblivious to his apnea, although he "felt terrible" all day. "Then my wife changed her job and sleeping pattern and started to notice that I stopped breathing in my sleep." The noise was awful but having never heard of sleep apnea, she put up with it.

Eventually her concern and disturbed sleep drove her to the edge and she finally put it to him "either breathe or leave." After two years of CPAP therapy he feels "like a million bucks."

On a recent visit he summed it up like this: "She doesn't mind the machine at all. In fact, it is so quiet compared to before the machine, it actually helps her sleep. The machine was like marriage counseling, I got my wife and my life back."

Things to Worry About After You Turn Off Late-Night Television

David Letterman's "Top Ten Lists" have been a staple for sleep-disordered Americans for more than a decade. With apologies to Letterman, here is my list of physical contributors to apnea (drawing on the levels of disordered breathing described in Chapter 5) based on my experiences with patients. I wish it could be funny.

10. Level-2 (palate) blockage.
9. "Kissing" tonsils (not common in adults).
8. A tongue that is too large for the lower jaw.
7. Small lower jaw with blockage that occurs in only one position, such as sleeping on your back.
6. Narrowing at any level combined with another acquired medical condition such as heart or lung disease.
5. Narrow airway at all levels that function well by day but close down at night after drinking alcohol, taking medication, or having an allergic reaction during sleep.
4. Severe allergies with polyps totally blocking level-1 nasopharynx.
3. A combination of nasal allergies with a hardware problem such as a long palate or a "software" (soft-tissue) problem such as a big tongue.
2. Level-3 "hardware" (bone structure) crowding, leading to a general traffic jam of soft tissue.

And by far the number one physical indicator of sleep apnea is:

1. Genetically programmed obstruction with obesity, a short neck, small lower jaw, and a combination of allergy-caused or structural nasal blockage and elongated soft palate.

7

SNORING AND APNEA TREATMENT

All treatment of snoring and obstruction to airflow, as in apnea, is based on the goal of clearing the way for air to flow from the nose and mouth to the lungs. If that airflow passes over excessive or floppy tissue but is not blocked outright, it results in vibration of the tissues, which produces the sound known as snoring. If the passage becomes narrow enough so that the flow of air is almost completely blocked or blocked entirely, it results in obstructed breathing or apnea.

Clearing the Upper Airways—Your Body in the Driver's Seat

Since snoring and apnea involve the same structures along the airway from nose and mouth to lungs, many of the treatments are the same. (To picture the shared anatomy and structures involved in both snoring and apnea, please refer to the diagram of the upper airway on page 66 and 78, in Chapter 5.)

To review briefly, level 1 problems are the ones in the nose and sinuses, such as nasal polyps, and allergies. Level 2 refers to problems of the palate being enlarged or swollen, uvula being enlarged, the tonsils, and the part of the tongue you can see. Level 3 refers to the back of tongue, the lower jaw, and inside or around the neck.

Throughout this chapter I will refer to those three anatomic levels of the upper airway and outline treatment for each level. I'll discuss available treatments for snoring and/or apnea for each anatomic level.

Snoring

Picture yourself on a long drive. Are there bends in the road where you have to slow down? Do you wish that highway engineers would straighten the road? Do trees ever get blown over in a high wind, forcing you to drive around them? Do storm drains ever overflow and flood the road? Is there construction that forces three lanes of traffic into one lane? Every time you encounter another obstacle, your patience goes down and your blood pressure goes up.

Do you suffer in silence when a half-hour drive turns into an hour or more? No. You curse. You complain to your passengers. You pound the steering wheel. You honk your horn. Your car is also suffering. That wear and tear is costing you money in both lousy gas mileage and long-term maintenance on the brakes and steering.

When you snore or have apnea, your body is going through similar stress. It's telling you to fix the potholes, get a tune-up, and get on with life. Listen to it!

The goal should be to reduce noise and vibration wherever it occurs before it damages other, currently healthy tissue. Remember the vacuum cleaner analogy from Chapter 5? It points out that normal air movement through an unobstructed vacuum cleaner hose sounds very different from the snoring sound generated when something gets stuck in the attachment. The noise means that there is something wrong and we should always fix it by removing the obstruction. Otherwise the machine won't get the job done of cleaning our home, and we risk long-term damage to the machine itself. This same principle applies to the body—to the nervous system, the blocked or snoring airway, and to the heart.

Starting at the Nose

The nasal passages provide the first line of resistance to airflow during sleep. Fixed structural obstruction from deviated nasal septum, nasal polyps, or tumors can contribute to snoring.

Reversible or dynamic blockage such as the mucus that builds from allergic rhinitis, or the common cold, can also reduce the flow of air.

Whatever the cause of blockage during sleep, reduction of airflow through the nose may contribute to mouth breathing. With the open mouth and downward, backward movement of the lower jaw, the tongue separates from the roof of the mouth and moves backward toward the throat, blocking or narrowing the airway. If the airway is also narrowed by things such as obesity, certain medications, or the general shape of the jaw or face, this tongue movement will cause altered airflow, vibration, and snoring or the more serious obstructive sleep apnea.

Anatomic Level-1 Treatment Options
ALLERGIC RHINITIS

Local nasal sprays and allergy pills may be very effective in reducing swelling. Nasal sprays may contain decongestants, antihistamines, steroids, and saline solution (salt water) in any combination. Pills designed to enter the blood system and travel to the blood vessels in the nasopharynx contain combinations of anti-inflammatories such as acetominophen or aspirin, decongestants, and antihistamines. The obvious difference is that sprays are topical, meaning they go directly on the inside tissues of the nose, while pills get there and everywhere else along the way, by the bloodstream. The manner in which the drugs are taken can have side effects, which are discussed below.

Decongestant sprays offer immediate relief, and many of them are available over the counter. However, don't confuse easy availability and fast relief with safety. They can cause lasting damage. This is especially true for those who have sleep-disordered breathing, since so many of you may also have heart conditions, diabetes, or other serious medical problems that require prescription medication. The medications you take for those conditions may result in dangerous interactions when used with decongestants in any form. Also, decongestants should be used very carefully, if at all, by pregnant or breast-feeding women, and by small children, and always under a doctor's care. There are three commonly used decongestants:

1. **Oxymetazoline** works by shrinking blood vessels in your body. The nasal sprays act directly on the blood vessels in your nasal tissues allowing them to drain, thus decreasing congestion. Nasal sprays that contain oxymetazoline include:

Afrin, Afrin Nasal Sinus, Allerest 12 Hour Nasal Spray, Neo-Synephrine 12 Hour, and many others.

Some of these medications, such as Neo-Synephrine and Afrin, may be habit forming. They may also keep you awake.

2. **Pseudoephedrine** is also available over the counter in tablets, capsules, extended-release (long-acting) tablets and capsules, liquid form, and drops for children. As the name implies, this is a synthetic form of ephedrine, which may act as a stimulant, so to avoid sleeping problems, take the last dose of the day several hours before bedtime. In some people, it may cause drowsiness. Follow the directions on the package label or on your prescription label carefully, and ask your doctor or pharmacist to explain any part you do not understand. Take pseudoephedrine exactly as directed.

3. **Phenylephrine** is used for temporary relief of nasal congestion caused by hay fever or other allergies, colds, or sinus trouble. It may also be used in ear infections to relieve congestion. It is found in Neo-Synephrine Nasal Spray, Neo-Synephrine Nasal Drops, Vicks Sinex, among many other medications.

Another decongestant, one that is low-tech and extremely low in price, is normal saline, also known as salt water. How does it work? When you have allergic rhinitis, the allergic swelling narrows your nasal passages and makes it harder for the air to flow in and out. Allergists recommend that you irrigate your nasal passages with what they call *hypertonic* saline solutions, which means they have a much higher salt concentration—2 to 3 percent—than the fluids in body tissues. (Most over-the-counter nasal sprays have an *isotonic* solution, which has a concentration equal to that in the body.) The greater concentration of salt draws moisture out of the swollen nasal passages into the mucous membranes through the lining of the airway by osmosis. This not only widens the nasal passages by reducing swelling, but helps restore the membranes' natural irrigating function. It keeps them moist and allows them to trap allergens before they penetrate deeper into the airways where they can trigger allergic or asthma attacks. After they are trapped by the moist mucus, they can be removed from the body by blowing your nose.

Home Remedy

This salt solution recipe comes from ENT specialists: one quart of tap water, two to three heaping teaspoons of sea salt or kosher salt (both have no additives) and one level teaspoon of baking soda. It can be administered using a 30 cc bulb syringe, which can be purchased at a pharmacy, to regulate dosing of your homemade version. Use as needed. It keeps indefinitely. Saline solutions can also be purchased in hypertonic strength over the counter. Saltaire is one such product, which comes in a plastic bottle ready made for spraying.

ANTIHISTAMINES

These drugs interfere with the release of a substance called histamine—one of a number of so-called mediators that are released by cells circulating in your bloodstream waiting to respond to the introduction of the things you are allergic to. Allergy reactions are really produced when a part of the immune system that was created to do one thing—defend your ancestors against organisms that they are no longer exposed to—goes looking for something else to do. We need histamine. It is one of the chemicals in your body that seems to be involved in controlling sleep and wakefulness. (You will read more about histamine and other chemicals that control the critical neuropathways in Chapter 8.) When you are awake, more histamine is being produced in your brain than when you are asleep, so naturally, the levels should fall at night, and normally they do.

However, if you are allergic to something in your bedroom, such as the dust in your bedding, your histamine levels will rise at the wrong time for a good night's sleep. Not only does this have a stimulative effect on your brain, but the allergic response in your airways can result in swelling of the tissues along the airways, which will narrow them and make snoring worse when you are asleep. If you have nasal allergies, you might take an antihistamine before you go to bed.

The older first-generation antihistamines, such as Benadryl, are available without prescription, and they may help you sleep because they cross the brain blood barrier and neutralize the histamine in your brain. Unfortunately, that makes them unsuitable for use during the day. In addition, there are other unwanted side effects such as morning hangover and dry mouth. They also may cause men to retain urine. These side effects make them less-than-optimal sleeping aids. Second-generation antihistamines, most of which are still by prescription only, do not usually have a sedative effect and work very well to reduce allergy-related snoring.

All the treatments discussed above can be used alone or in combination to reduce swollen tissues and symptoms related to snoring and obstructive sleep apnea. The treatments, including normal saline, should be used only short-term and under medical direction.

Immunotherapy desensitization. This treatment is known popularly as allergy shots. By regularly introducing small amounts of the substances you are allergic to into your system, the allergist is retraining your immune system not to react to these allergens. This method is effective in 60 to 70 percent of cases, but it works only after prolonged treatment.

Environmental cleanup. Houses are full of allergens, such as dust. Your bedroom particularly is an allergen farm. Dust mites thrive on dead skin, and your mattress is full of both. Thorough cleaning, regular laundering of bedclothes and an air purification system with a HEPA (high-efficiency purification apparatus) filter may be very effective for cleaning the air. And don't let your pets sleep with you!

BE PREPARED

If you are allergic to, say, cats or dogs and you are planning to spend time with a friend who has one, you can prepare yourself well in advance and thus avoid staying up all night sneezing and wheezing by taking a drug called cromolyn sodium, which is sold over the counter under the name NasalCrom. It is incredibly safe and helps stave off allergic reactions when taken before high exposure to allergens by in effect gumming up the cells that release histamine.

Fixed Blockages
NASAL VALVE DILATION

The nasal valve is the narrowed part of the upper airway, just above the nares, and it is prone to blockage. There are basically two kinds of nasal valve dilators. The first are those adhesive strips that football players wear over the bridge of the nose. You will apply these at bedtime. These strips cost about 80 cents each and cannot be reused.

The Breathe Right Strip is an example of an adhesive nasal strip. Many of my patients report satisfaction with them, and—I confess—I use them. However, they won't work if the nose is congested, if there are generalized allergies, or if there is in obstruction downstream in the air tubes.

Occasional problems include irritation of the skin, especially in those with sensitive skin, and that the strips sometimes come off in the middle of the night.

The second type of nasal valve dilator is an internal splint. This is usually a flexible plastic strip that is designed for actual insertion into the nostrils at night. However, they are enormously problematic and I have never recommended using them. They cost anywhere from $20 to $30 each and have to be replaced several times a year. As you might imagine, they can also be rather uncomfortable and when used regularly may cause breakdown or irritation of the inside lining of the nose.

NOSE FOR THE FUTURE

The nose is the front door for normal air movement and I believe we need more low-tech ways to treat blockage at this level, without resorting to medication or surgery. Unfortunately, nasal valve dilators are reported to be useful in only 5 to 10 percent of patients who snore or have apnea.

There might be other ways to treat nasal obstructions mechanically. The challenge, however, lies in doing it *comfortably*. The nose is a complex structure designed not only to allow air to move but to filter it. The tissues inside the nose are sensitive, and they are supposed to be. When something enters the nostrils that is not supposed to be there, you sneeze.

If your nose feels blocked when you breathe through it and does not feel clearer with allergy treatment or breathing strips, there may be a more serious blockage. This requires a visit to your doctor or an ENT specialist for further review and probable evaluation of the total upper airway, nose to vocal cords, with a special light called a fiberscope.

DEVIATED SEPTUM OR POLYPS

Any fixed blockage along the airway, from the tip of the nose to the tip of the palate (or roof of the mouth) can contribute to snoring or apnea.

If the problem is clearly identified after careful screening as being related to an obvious fixed structural or hardware problem, then nasal surgery is indicated. If, for example, the problem is a severely deviated septum, which is a bend in the cartilage that separates your nasal passages, it will have to be straightened. If there are polyps, growths, blocking the passages themselves, they will have to be removed.

If such surgery is indicated, preoperative evaluation and screening for other related conditions are mandatory. Your family doctor must be involved at all steps of the planned surgery. A careful review of symptoms before the surgery will determine the need for further testing, such as a sleep study, or other treatments. Many insurance companies now request a sleep study prior to approving any ENT surgery when snoring is accompanied by symptoms and/or findings of apnea.

Anatomic Level-2 and-3 Treatments (Dental Appliances)

Dental or oral appliances are special mouthpieces fashioned by a dentist or orthodontist to fit your teeth and jaw. Dental appliances have been used to treat bruxism, or teeth grinding, and temporomandibular joint (TMJ) problems. They are very useful in treating snoring and some cases of sleep apnea.

HOW DO THESE DEVICES WORK TO PREVENT SNORING?

Snoring occurs when air moves between or around crowded or swollen tissue in the air passage during sleep. As the person breathes, the tissues of the throat start to vibrate. The main culprits are the soft palate (which includes the uvula and the tongue) and crowding caused by the bony structures of the face (mandible and maxilla). Dental appliances work by opening up the back of the throat so that the vibrating tissues are kept apart, thus making it easier for the air to flow.

There are many oral appliances available over the counter and an even larger number on the Internet. However, the only two types approved by the FDA at this time are mandibular advancing devices, which move the lower jaw forward, and tongue-retaining devices, which allow the tongue to move forward away from the back of the throat, but not backward.

Both devices require a special fitting of a moldable material designed to fit over the teeth and change the shape or position of the hardware (teeth and jawbone position) or software (palate and tongue). Actual fitting and fabrication may take several visits. This follow-up is necessary to make final adjustments and to screen for possible complications or side affects.

The mandibular advancing device not only moves the lower jaw forward; it pulls the tongue along with it, creating even more space for air to move freely along the back of the throat. Refer again to the picture on page 71. The last panel on the right shows crowding of the airway due to a disproportionately small lower jaw. The mandibular advancing device corrects this by moving the jaw forward clearing the airway.

The tongue-retaining device is the second type of oral appliance. It is a mouthpiece that allows a space for the tongue to move forward past the teeth with a slightly opened mouth, thus clearing the way for air to move along the back of the throat.

The decision to use an oral appliance and the actual fitting and follow-up is fairly complicated. Any such decision will require discussion between you and your sleep doctor, ENT specialist, orthodontist, dentist, or general practitioner.

Most professionals evaluating a patient for an oral appliance insist on a sleep study first. A careful sleep history review and physical evaluation and, when indicated, a sleep study are the only ways to determine whether a patient snores or has a more serious apnea.

Severity alert! Although an excellent option for some patients who snore, appliances by themselves are appropriate only for those with mild or moderate apnea and only in selected cases. They should not be the sole method of treating severe sleep apnea. As with any treatment option, a follow-up sleep study may be necessary if symptoms continue.

Cost. The price can range from $50 to $2,000. The cheaper devices can be plucked off a shelf at a drugstore and be potentially harmful if you have apnea or a more severe breathing disorder. In fact, the Food and Drug Administration (FDA) has issued an Internet warning for all such devices, citing the dangers associated with untreated sleep apnea.

On the other end of the spectrum thousands of dollars can be spent on testing, X rays of the jaw, teeth, and airway, and the eventual purchase of a custom-fitted higher-end oral appliance. The extra cost features may include, for example, a tiny built-in adjustable screw that allows week-by-week adjustment with minimal discomfort.

Comfort. Devices that move the lower jaw forward are usually more comfortable than those that reposition the tongue. Custom-made appliances using high-quality materials that mold more securely and precisely are generally are more comfortable than those made of cheaper materials. The more natural-fitting and less bulky the better.

Durability. Over-the-counter devices generally last less than one year. Custom-made appliances require periodic adjustment and may last for many years.

Adjustability and mobility. Less expensive devices usually have only one size and setting. One size definitely does not fit all! Some, but not all, custom-made devices can be adjusted so that the right amount of jaw advancement is set or horizontal and vertical motion can be varied. The high-end variety may be necessary in patients with preexisting or newly developed TMJ or other jaw problems.

Some devices are marketed to be fitted at home using heat labile plastics that mold into place. Others allow self-adjustments. Considering the potential for incorrect fit or inadequate treatment of a more serious condition such as apnea, it is preferable to have a certified dentist or orthodontist approve use of the device and make the adjustments to ensure maximum comfort and effectiveness. The newly formed Dental Sleep Society is an organization dedicated to continued education and quality care in this area. (See resources, page 295.)

If you have a lot of dental work, consult with your dentist about the use of these devices since they can cause damage or shifting to your bridgework. Some of the components may cause an allergic reaction in susceptible individuals.

Despite the challenges, dental or oral appliances are easy to use and maintain. The better models are adjustable and, of course, very portable. As with any device or appliance close follow-up with a qualified specialist gives the most bang for the buck and greatest chance of successful treatment.

SURGERY FOR LEVEL-2 SNORING

Oropharynx Surgery

Oropharynx surgery describes any procedure that reduces the size of the redundant or excessive soft tissue of the upper airway, or makes that tissue more rigid and therefore less likely to vibrate, which will reduce the noise of snoring. This can be palate and uvula surgery or surgery on the other parts of the pharynx or both: thus the name uvulopalatopharyngoplasty, or UPPP for short. Essentially the surgery involves removing the extra tissue from the palate or around the tonsils so that the back of the throat is widened, allowing more air to move and reducing snoring and apnea. The surgery can be done with a regular scalpel or with lasers. The side effects include short-term pain and a change in the way you swallow.

The most challenging problem with palate surgery is to determine who will benefit from it. More and more insurance companies are insisting on a sleep study prior to approving payment for palate or airway surgery to correct snoring, which is a good thing. ENT specialists or surgeons will tell you that the success rate for correcting snoring or apnea is high, but only when the tissue causing the snoring is easily identified.

Unfortunately, when snoring or apnea occurs because of several areas of narrowing or swelling along the airway, as it often does, a single surgical procedure may not stop the problem. In fact, if you have several sites of obstruction such as the nasopharynx and behind the tongue, a single-palate surgery may fail to correct the problem. The nose and the base of the tongue continue to block the airway and the typical response is "Why did I bother?" The failures tend to be related not to failed surgery but to obstructions at other levels or to additional conditions such as obesity.

Several studies have been done to find other ways to shrink or stiffen the enlarged palate. For example, in radiofrequency ablation, a needle is inserted into the palate in several locations at a high enough frequency to essentially microwave a piece of tissue in the palate about the size of a small marble. The tissue is intended to scar as it heals, and thereby shrink and stiffen.

Another technique developed by the Army involves injecting the uvula with a liquid called tetradecyl sulfate, a chemical that causes a type of cell death and scarring called sclerosis. This sclerosing agent has been used for some time to treat varicose veins. One of several problems with these injections is the potential for a severe allergic reaction, which is not something you want when you are trying to keep your airway clear.

WHAT YOU CAN'T HEAR CAN STILL HURT YOU

Important as it is to reduce or eliminate snoring, the problems may not end when the noise stops. As mentioned above in the discussion of palate surgery, successful snoring treatment may miss apnea. As I tell my patients, "You can take the rattle out of the rattlesnake, but it can still bite you."

This is why a sleep study, or at the very least a very thorough screening by your doctor or a sleep specialist, prior to surgery is so important. This is not excessive, expensive "defensive medicine" but good, sound medical practice, and most insurance companies recognize it. They know that a proper evaluation now will save them money in the long run in outlays for treatment of chronic medical conditions. If there is snoring with no apnea or minimal apnea, a carefully planned and targeted surgery can be sufficient. If there is a mild or moderate level of sleep apnea, surgery may also be sufficient, or it might be combined with an oral appliance or other treatment such as CPAP. However, for snoring associated with severe apnea, surgery is rarely used as a first step in treatment except in unusual cases such as a definite level-1 blockage from a large tumor or where the anatomy is clearly in the way. Surgery becomes a more viable option for moderate or severe sleep apnea when other methods cannot be used or are not tolerated. Otherwise, there is no reason not to use CPAP in the vast majority of cases of severe obstructive sleep apnea. Surgery, even "minor" surgery, is a serious decision to make, and you should consider all your options before committing to any treatment plans.

Treatment of Obstructive Sleep Apnea Syndrome (All Levels—1, 2, and 3)
CPAP

CPAP stands for continuous positive airway pressure. It is the main treatment for obstructive sleep apnea syndrome and several other breathing disorders during sleep. The concept of delivering air under pressure through a hose and mask attached to the face is about 20 years old. Previously, severe obstructive sleep apnea was best treated with a tracheostomy, which obviously is pretty drastic.

The first CPAP machines used a motor like the one in a vacuum cleaner attached to a hose. It was fastened to the patient's face using a moldable Silastic material to hold it in place. The mask is also known as the interface. CPAP worked by pushing air through the air passage at a pressure high enough to keep the soft airways from collapsing. It is essentially an air splint for the entire airway.

After about five years of successful use, the mechanical blower, mask, and associated gadgets were developed enough to allow CPAP to enter mainstream treatment as an alternative to a tracheotomy. CPAP has improved significantly since its invention in 1980. Today there are so many models of both the machine and mask that I am constantly getting calls from patients who are confused about their options. Today a typical machine looks like this:

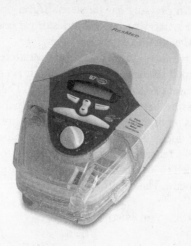

©Resmed 2004. Used with permission.

The CPAP is a medical device and as such all models must be approved by the FDA before going on sale. Although they are available on the Internet you must have a physician's prescription in order to obtain a CPAP. Use caution when buying over the Internet since things like supplies or maintenance costs may offset the initial bargain. There may also be a problem with warranties. Your insurance company will either rent the device or pay for purchasing the device from a DME, or *durable medical equipment,* company. All DME companies request a copy of the sleep study results along with the doctor's prescription at the time of the CPAP order.

If you want a specific brand or type of CPAP with added features, you can communicate directly with the DME company about your needs. If you are not satisfied with what the DME company tells you, check with your insurance carrier about options, including contacting another company. The DME company should arrange a visit to the home for first-time users. This visit includes a safety inspection of the vicinity where you will be using the machine and suggestions as to the best location for setting it up. During that same visit, you'll get instructions on using CPAP and making adjustments to the fit of the mask. Finally, the maintenance schedule is reviewed, with details on filter hose and mask changes and humidifier upkeep.

In addition to the standard options including carrying case, color, and humidifier, you can ask about "ramp" features, which will time a gradual increase in pressure as you sleep. Travel options can include alternative power sources such as batteries or car converter. Machines can be very lightweight and extremely quiet.

A bilevel positive airway pressure machine is different from the CPAP in that it is designed to deliver two different air pressures, one for the breath in and a lower pressure for the breath out. This may help you tolerate the air pressure better than a CPAP at a high setting. Since the bilevel machine is more expensive than a CPAP, it requires justification from the treating doctor. Other models have compliance monitors built in, which internally record the hours of proper usage. This information can be downloaded to an analysis and reporting program for a focused review by your doctor. These features are discussed in more detail below.

THE CPAP MASK—THE "SHOE" THAT FITS

The CPAP mask attaches you to your CPAP machine. This is also called the interface, as mentioned above. The mask comes in more shapes and sizes than you see at a Halloween party. These include nasal pillows, nasal masks, nose and mouth masks, and full face masks, to name a few. When you go to a shoe store, the things you focus on are comfort, style, and color; comfort is determined by the correct size and fit. CPAP mask sizes also sound like shoe sizes: small, medium wide, and extra large in all combinations. Like a pair of shoes, the best way to choose a mask is to try it on. In addition to many shapes and sizes, they also have a variety of straps and headgear to hold them in place. Since you move about in your sleep the mask and headgear should move with you and be easy to adjust. The tubing length cannot be too long, since there is a risk of a drop in pressure. After some trial and error, you will learn how to position the tube for maximal stability. You can also purchase special arms designed to hold the hose in an optimal position.

In recent years, shoes have been sold with a variety of cushioning materials to make them more comfortable. CPAP manufacturers have taken a page from the shoemaker's book. CPAP masks may be lined with a soft lining such as gels, foams, and even a balloonlike air interface for better comfort. Wound-healing films to help prevent skin irritation, adhesives, heat-labile molds, and special oral masks for those who cannot tolerate the nasal or oronasal masks are also available.

The most commonly used masks share the necessary design of fitting over the nose and/or mouth and having some way to attach it to the head:

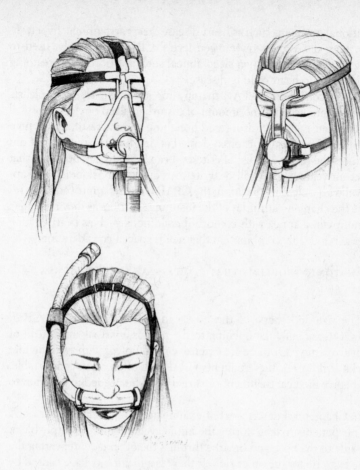

Adapted from Resmed 2004. Used with permission.

WHO SHOULD GET CPAP?

There are several reasons for recommending CPAP therapy. The most common is to treat significant sleep apnea based on the results of a sleep study. This could be moderate or severe apnea with or without complicating factors such as heart arrhythmias.

We also prescribe CPAP for less severe apnea when clinical observation suggests the need for it. For example, a patient with only mild apnea, based on the number of times they stop breathing every hour—12 times per hour on the breathing disorder index—would not qualify for CPAP according to Medicare guidelines unless the patient also has additional problems such as heart disease, heart arrhythmia, hypertension, lung disease, or low oxygen levels. CPAP can also be used to treat conditions other then sleep apnea, such as disordered breathing at night due to heart or lung disease.

When considering CPAP therapy for a patient, sleep specialists also take into account the amount of disturbed sleep or electrocortical arousals caused by the disordered breathing and the resulting daytime sleepiness. The request is often denied at first because the patient did not meet the recipe-like list of criteria. I can honestly say, however, that in recent years when I call or write to request reconsideration of approval with a clear justification, the CPAP is always approved. This reflects the changing attitudes of the insurance carriers as they recognize that untreated apnea with comorbid conditions such as heart or lung disease is a deadly combination that needs special consideration.

ANATOMIC PROBLEMS THAT COMPLICATE CPAP TREATMENT—
LEVEL 1

The size and shape of the nose can create problems for CPAP users. Occasionally the opening to the nose is a virtual slit instead of an oval opening. Or there are extensive nasal polyps with swelling that blocks airflow. For these patients CPAP will often be uncomfortable. Aggressive medical treatment or surgery will be needed in addition to CPAP.

In Chapter 5, I describe a self-examination step similar to the one I ask my patients to take during the initial evaluation. You simply block one side of the nose and breathe through the other side, repeating the same exercise for the other side. If there is a major blockage caused by a hardware problem such as a severe narrowing from a deviated nasal septum or tumor, CPAP probably will not work well. If no blockage is suggested by a focused review of the medical history or none is found on the initial physical examination, then you are cleared to try CPAP if needed.

Even if there is no obvious blockage, however, problems can develop as air flows in and out of the nose during sleep. This can cause dryness or a reaction called vasoactive rhinitis. Vasoactive means blood vessel response and rhinitis means runny nose. We fix this by adding a humidifier to the CPAP machine, which adds moisture, sort of like an internal sauna or warm moist ocean breeze, or with use of short-term medication.

Active upper airway infection such as sinusitis or chronic sinusitis will create sensitive and swollen tissues that react with pain when pressure is applied. Report such pain or discomfort to your doctor. You may have to stay off CPAP until the condition is fully treated.

LEVEL-2 ANATOMIC PROBLEMS AND CPAP

Any large growth or tumor will interfere with the ability of CPAP to do its job. I have seen walnut-sized tumors that caused sleep apnea that CPAP could not push past. Once the tumor was removed, the apnea responded to much lower levels of CPAP pressure, and in some cases the CPAP was discontinued altogether. Surgery is usually needed for very large adenoids or the so-called kissing tonsils, which are so large that they touch each other, totally blocking the airway, as well. Again, refer to the example of kissing tonsils, page 75.

ORAL APPLIANCE FOR APNEA

As mentioned above, an oral appliance can be used for level-2 or -3 obstructive apnea in combination with CPAP and other treatments.

LEVEL-3 ANATOMIC PROBLEMS AND CPAP

When the tongue is very large in proportion to the mouth cavity or when the lower jaw is very small and as a result pushes the tongue back against the airway, the CPAP setting may be uncomfortably high. In these cases, the mouth may also fly open and allow air to escape. In such cases, a strap designed to keep the chin in position may solve the problem.

When anatomy—bone structure, tongue position, or both—continues to present a problem, a combination of therapies may prove very helpful. In such cases, an oral appliance can be added to the CPAP treatment to help move the large tongue or small lower jaw out of the way. There is a company that makes a single device containing a nasal pillow CPAP mask attached to the oral appliance. The advantage is that the jaw and tongue are moved forward by a mouthpiece that doubles as an anchor for the CPAP hose and the pillows that cushion the face. There is no need for additional headgear to hold the pillows in place.

About 20 percent of patients have difficulty with the CPAP machine. This is not surprising since the patient is, in effect, learning a new way to sleep after a lifetime of "doing what comes naturally." Sleep centers always take steps to help patients adjust to this change. There is an educational session during every initial visit where we explain the operation of the device, show a video and/or pictures, and answer questions about CPAP operation and maintenance. If there is a level of anxiety that interferes with CPAP usage, the patient will be invited to the lab during the day to give it a test run. This session includes a mask fitting. My own approach is to compare CPAP to buying a pair of shoes, as I explained earlier. Just as it is very difficult to look at a shoe and predict how it is going to feel on your foot when you walk, the same is true for a CPAP mask. We are successful in persuading almost 50 percent of the initial nonbelievers to use a mask. And once they do give it a try, they are generally convinced.

PITFALLS

Mask Too Tight or Marks on the Face?

As with a pair of shoes, a mask may be too tight and mark the face. You may have the wrong style mask for the shape of your face, which might prompt you to tighten the straps too much. Or you may have an inflammatory reaction caused by sensitive skin or being allergic to one of the components in the mask. In such cases you should not hesitate to call the DME company (the phone number should be on the side of the machine or in your paperwork) or you can call your physician. For difficult-to-solve or more serious problems we invite patients back to the sleep center for a visit.

Mask Falls Off in the Middle of the Night?

This is a common complaint. The mask may come off in response to excessive movement or when the pressure setting is too low or too high. You will soon become adept at adjusting the mask quickly and going back to sleep. Assuming the mask is a good fit, things will improve in time. You may want to experiment with different straps or try a different mask if the problem continues. In the event that you have a large weight change or another major change in your airway, or anatomy, you may want to revisit your doctor and discuss recalibrating the CPAP.

The Pressure Is Too High

If the CPAP pressure is high or you are very sensitive to it, you may need a "ramp" feature, previously mentioned, which allows you to fall asleep with the pressure at a low level but then very slowly increasing until the final setting is reached. On occasion I cannot help the patient tolerate CPAP and in that case will go to the bilevel machine discussed earlier. Instead of full and steady pressure while inhaling and exhaling, the bilevel gives a full pressure as you breathe in and then cuts the pressure to a lower number as you breathe out. Like trying to walk up a down escalator, breathing out against high pressure requires more effort than many of us can comfortably deal with.

COMPLIANCE

As with any other form of long-term medical treatment, using CPAP requires conscientious use. A diabetic has to take his or her insulin; a heart attack patient with heart disease must stick to diet and exercise regimens as well as prescribed courses of medication, and so on. CPAP is like that. Yet, as with these other conditions, there's a tendency to equate relief with cure. That's an illusion. One longtime CPAP user stepped on his mask and broke it. He had been feeling so good for so long that he didn't replace it right away. Within the space of a week, he fell asleep on the job, and this was witnessed by a supervisor. Fortunately, with treatment and a letter from the sleep center, he returned to work happier and healthier.

Still, for some people, the simple act of compliance is not enough. The therapy may be working, but it may engender a new problem—insomnia. No one wants to lie in bed wide awake with a machine attached to his or her face. For these people, an additional course of behavioral therapy, guided imagery, and even medications, all of which you will read about in Chapter 10, are sometimes needed to help with CPAP compliance.

Finally, not all that snores is apnea. Tumors, infections, and weak muscles in the area of the vocal cords and surrounding structures can cause a snoring noise when breathing in. CPAP therapy may actually be harmful in some of these conditions. Discuss any discomfort caused by the CPAP with your doctor.

Surgery on the Lower Jaw for Apnea (Anatomic Level 3)

This is advanced surgery and reserved for severe cases where CPAP isn't tolerated. It requires a special team of highly skilled surgeons and specialists and therefore cannot be done at every sleep center.

One procedure involves reconstructive surgery on the jawbone, which actually moves the jaw forward and brings the tongue and other structures with it. This is called mandibular advancement and it is usually reserved for patients with a severely deficient lower jaw (known as a retroplaced mandible). A sign of a retroplaced mandible may be a severe overbite where the upper teeth are farther forward than the lower teeth.

The jaw is usually wired shut after this surgery to allow healing. Postoperative complications may include a problem with misalignment of teeth and numbness related to small nerve damage. Nonetheless, I have seen dramatic improvements in the apnea and in the general appearance of patients after this surgery. Better looks and better sleep—can't beat that.

Tongue Surgery for Apnea

In most cases of severe apnea the back of the tongue is the last possible blockage point, and the most crucial and most overlooked. You can fix the nose and shrink the palate and the back of the tongue can still block the airway. Refer to level 3 on pages 66 and 78.

Plastic surgery on the tongue to remove or shrink a portion of the back of the tongue can allow more air movement and reduce apnea. However, patients must be carefully selected because the potential effects on the ability to eat and speak can be significant and troubling.

Body Position Therapy for Snoring and Apnea

As I pointed out earlier, the voluntary muscles relax during sleep and particularly during REM sleep. The tongue is one of those. In that relaxed state, it very commonly will block the back of the throat, especially when you are lying on your back in deep or REM sleep or basking in the afterglow of a good Barolo. When a sleep study shows that apnea or snoring only happen when you are on your back, the condition is called "supine" or "on-your-back" disordered breathing.

Treatments for this type of snoring or apnea are much lower-tech than surgery.

One patient returned to me after following my instructions, thrilled that she had had her first good night's sleep in years. The miracle cost her $1.98 plus tax. It consisted of some safety pins and three tennis balls purchased at a 99 cent store. At my direction, she inserted three tennis balls into separate socks and pinned them to the back of her nightshirt at the level of her shoulder blades. "I didn't have to buy the socks. Every time I do the laundry, at least one comes back without its mate. They just pile up in the laundry room. Now I can recycle them."

There are more sophisticated pillows and harnesses available in stores and on the Internet, but basically they do the same thing as the tennis balls. They keep you off your back so you don't snore or choke on your tongue.

For patients who are very obese, sleeping with the head of the bed elevated to at least 30 degrees relieves the pressure on the diaphragm from the abdomen and may facilitate air movement at the back of the throat. Some patients have developed the habit of sleeping facedown. However, this can place strain on the neck and lower back and may interfere with air movement in and out of the lungs.

Avoid Alcohol and Sedatives

This applies to snoring and apnea and has been covered in other chapters. Any substance that causes muscle tone to decrease will worsen snoring and apnea.

The Most Difficult Treatment of All

Hardly a day goes by when we don't hear a story about the obesity epidemic in the United States. In 1991, four states reported obesity rates of 15 to 19 percent and nine states reported rates at or above 20 percent.

By 2002, 20 states had obesity rates of 15 to 19 percent; 29 states had rates of 20 to 24 percent; and one state reported a rate over 25 percent.

The villains are well-known—supersized fast-food portions and lack of exercise, soda vending machines, and hours spent cruising the Internet and watching television.

Obesity is an important risk factor for apnea—studies show that 60 percent of people with apnea are significantly overweight. It is a factor in snoring as well. However, rather substantial weight loss—15 to 30 percent—is often required to produce a significant reduction in symptoms. This can be very difficult to achieve, considering a success rate of 5 to 15 percent for most weight loss programs.

Because drugs can cause other problems, they are used sparingly for treating obesity. Medications may be effective, however, when used under the direct and careful supervision of a physician familiar with this type of therapy.

Weight Loss Surgery

In cases of severe life-threatening obesity, gastric bypass (gastro-plasty or bariatric surgery) can result in dramatic weight loss, which then helps reduce apnea and disordered breathing both day and night, and improves health in general. The surgery is not indicated for snor-ing alone and since it is associated with possible complications should only be performed at specialized centers.

The many celebrities who have undergone gastroplasty have popu-larized this approach. But there is no magic to it, and it should be per-formed only when the patient's life is at stake and after a thorough evaluation and attempts to treat the condition medically.

I am on a team that evaluates gastroplasty candidates at the New York Methodist Hospital, with weight reduction problems. Approximately 60 percent of those patients with morbid obesity have obstructive sleep ap-nea. For every 22 pounds gained, the risk of sleep apnea doubles. For every five-inch increase in waist size, the risk quadruples. The majority of gastroplasty candidates have several other weight-related problems such as hip- and knee-joint disease, hypertension, and diabetes. Some studies show the life span of a morbidly obese person may be reduced by 10–20 years. Even with risks like these, we are very cautious with the use of gas-troplasty. The procedure is only approved as a life-extending treatment after intensive testing, and failed behavioral therapies.

Sleep Medicine and Weight Loss Medicine Have Much in Common

A multidisciplinary approach to weight loss is still absent from most medical training programs. Doctors will treat hypertension and diabetes but only advise patients in passing about losing weight.

Sound familiar? It should. As I said in the Introduction, sleep dis-orders have long been viewed by most physicians as isolated nighttime problems with no urgent connection to the diseases they treat during the day.

Eating and exercising are, to be sure, wake time activities, but the process of weight gain continues even when you are asleep. You don't gain 10 pounds in a week only when your eyes are open! You read in the discussion of sleep hygiene about how long before bedtime to eat, how to get a good night's sleep, and what kinds of things you should eat. And you have read about the circadian clock for internal functions, such as glandular activity. Respecting your body during sleep means not overloading on the wrong kind of food. A proper diet can help you lose weight in your sleep, and the wrong types of food before bedtime will set the stage for weight gain during sleep.

In treating weight gain, as with so many other medical conditions, doctors who treat daytime diseases have common cause with sleep medicine. Fortunately, weight reduction medicine is now beginning to get the kind of attention that sleep medicine has also received with the addition of multidisciplinary training at many medical schools. In my own hospital, we have added a clinic for weight loss. Considering how long excessive weight has been recognized as a risk factor for our health, it is fairly surprising that this has not happened sooner. But better late than never.

You now know that snoring is no laughing matter. It places physical stress on your body, and physical and mental stress on those around you. Severe snoring can be seen as the most "contagious" form of a breathing disorder during sleep . . . you end up sharing your misery. Worse, snoring is often a predictor of sleep apnea, the impact of which may be so severe that it is literally killing you a little bit every time you go to sleep. The bad news is these disorders, without treatment, are not likely to go away by themselves. The good news is that treatment is effective, and readily available. If you are one of the millions of people suffering, either directly or indirectly, from snoring or sleep apnea, see your doctor or a sleep specialist. You don't have to live with these conditions; there is help.

NARCOLEPSY—WHEN SLEEP "ATTACKS"

In his 1963 autobiography, *How to Talk Dirty and Influence People,* comedian Lenny Bruce described a condition that had afflicted him since his wartime service in the U.S. Navy, which he attributed to a severe case of hepatitis. He was "plagued for many years with spells of lethargy," which were so severe they could be called "attacks."

He wrote: "I would find myself simultaneously dictating and sleeping—and since I speak in a stream of conscious[ness], apparently unrelated pattern, secretaries would be typing into eight-ten [*sic*] minutes of mumbling and abstraction, such as one might expect from a half-awake, half-asleep reporter."

After falling asleep one afternoon while driving and waking up in a ditch, he decided to consult a doctor, who queried him about a history of narcolepsy. The doctor "prescribed an amphetamine, which I believe is the generic term for Dexedrine, Benzedrine, Byphetamine, and the base for most diet pills, mood elevators, pep pills, thrill pills, etc."

For anyone who knows Bruce's history of drug abuse, that period in his life might have been the beginning of a perilous and finally fatal journey.

"Seized by Sleepiness"

One of the things that makes Bruce's story stand out is that the diagnosis of narcolepsy was considered at a time when the condition was so little understood. Narcolepsy in conjunction with cataplexy, a condition you will read about shortly, was first identified as a medical disorder in 1877. The word *narcolepsy* is from the Greek and means "seized by sleepiness," which sums up most of what we knew about it until comparatively recently. Taking a cue from the burgeoning field of psychosexuality, early theories associated narcolepsy with psychological problems. Somewhat later, when psychoanalytic explanations for medical problems were popular, there was a theory that narcolepsy was a form of "escape." Treating the condition on an analyst's couch must have been interesting since the patient would probably fall asleep right away and stay asleep for most of the appointment.

Narcolepsy was often wrongly diagnosed among women. Complaints that we currently recognize as narcolepsy were attributed to hysteria, depression, and hypoglycemia, among other disorders—which, when we consider what we now know about narcolepsy, that it affects women and men in equal numbers, possibly reflects the prevalent biases about women of the day.

Whatever the precise source of the condition, today we understand that narcolepsy is a neurological disorder involving abnormal episodes of REM sleep, disturbed sleep, and excessive sleepiness during the day. While we have made breakthroughs in our understanding of narcolepsy since the discovery of REM sleep in the early 1950s, just a few years after Lenny Bruce began to experience symptoms, 50 years later there are still many questions about its causes and treatment, although recent research suggests that narcolepsy may be related to destruction or alteration of a specific group of cells in the brain, which function as a kind of switch between the sleeping and waking states.

We know that narcolepsy can start at any age, although it frequently becomes noticeable in one's early 20s. The disorder is lifelong once it asserts itself, and a full set of symptoms may present themselves over time. Once the condition is established, however, it is not thought to be degenerative. That is, it usually does not worsen over time, in the way Parkinson's disease does, for example. Neither does it reduce one's life span. As you will read, the biochemistry of narcolepsy treatment is advancing, but as of yet there is no "cure."

Narcoleptic or Just Really Tired?

A bout of narcolepsy is sometimes referred to as a "sleep attack." This is a misleading term; it implies a normal wakeful state interrupted by an irresistible urge to sleep. Most of us have experienced this pressure after missing a night's sleep. My residents have been known to nod off during my lectures on narcolepsy, but only after an all-night hospital shift.

By contrast, people with full-blown narcolepsy do not have a normal waking state. Rather, their waking state is constantly opposed by pressure to sleep. If normal circadian rhythm is a succession of waves, as discussed in Chapters 2 and 3, the narcoleptic might be described as someone whose tide is trying to go in and out at the same time. Because of the development of the ability to track brain waves using EEG technology, we now understand that narcolepsy is typified by a faulty switch, as described above, between the waking and the sleep state, and most dramatically, between waking and REM sleep.

Escalating Symptoms

Full-blown narcolepsy usually develops over a long period of time. Because the symptoms do not set in all at once, the condition often goes undiagnosed for a decade. In the meantime, the accumulation of symptoms takes an escalating toll on a person's quality of life.

In cases of early narcolepsy, or evolving narcolepsy, the person will spend a normal amount of time in bed trying to sleep, although the quality of sleep will probably be disturbed to the point that they will feel additional sleep pressure during the day. In this respect, the problem will look like excessive daytime sleepiness, which, of course, can result from conditions other than narcolepsy.

Because of the increased pressure to sleep during the day and the fragmented, unsatisfactory nighttime sleep, there is a tendency to fall asleep at times that at first might seem unremarkable, such as during a boring lecture, while watching TV, or after a heavy lunch. Over time, however, these sleep episodes become a bit more conspicuous, such as dozing off during a meeting or during almost any quiet moment during the day. Still, this is not enough to diagnose narcolepsy, as you will read.

People who fall asleep in this fashion will often deny having a serious problem if they are confronted about their behavior. They will blame the occurrence on medication, illness, or some other temporary affliction. This state of denial can last indefinitely, until they find that their work performance, grades, or general quality of life is suffering.

As the symptoms mature, narcoleptic episodes can not only be embarrassing but debilitating and even dangerous to the sufferer and others. If you have seen the movie *Rat Race,* you will recall that the main character, played by Rowan Atkinson, actually fell asleep while walking. This is no exaggeration. People with narcolepsy fall asleep while eating, driving, and even swimming. Cats with narcolepsy will fall asleep with their face in their food. And in a couple one of whom is narcoleptic, the expression "sleep together" can mean one thing to one partner and something very different to the other—a narcoleptic can actually fall asleep during sexual intercourse.

States of Consciousness

At our current level of understanding, most of us exist in one of three states from some time before birth up until our physical death. As described in Chapter 2, we are either awake or in one of two states of sleep—REM or non-REM. While we think of the three states as separate, they probably coexist with one another, defining our behavior at predictable intervals throughout the 24-hour day. In the morning, most of us are awake and alert. At about three in the afternoon, there's sufficient pressure from the sleep state to convince many people to take a very civilized siesta, although most of the working world must fight the urge. For the most part, we stay in the wake state until it is time for bed.

Our bodies then shut down to a state that comes as close to what science fiction fans will recognize as suspended animation as we can get—during which we are capable of doing anything from reliving the previous day at work to taking a journey worthy of *Star Trek.* For those of us who don't think in science fiction terms, picture the photographs taken from space of the earth, half in light and half in darkness. Remember that just because half the world is in darkness, that doesn't mean it has ceased to function. Much of it is very busy. Likewise, with sleep, part of the brain is functioning on autopilot while another is actively orchestrating the trade-off between the oblivion of non-REM and the unbounded imagination of REM. If all goes well, the result of this nightly journey is nothing short of a mental and physical rebirth.

That's if all goes well.

But for one American out of 2,000, all does not go well. That is the rate at which we suffer from narcolepsy, which is about the same rate that we suffer from multiple sclerosis. For these people, life can be like a conversation rudely interrupted. They go from the waking state into a partial sleeping state, often without warning.

As stated above, because of the development of EEG technology, we can now track the functioning of the brain. This ability has allowed us to perceive symptoms of narcolepsy as the intrusion of non-REM sleep and REM sleep into wakefulness, and the intrusion of awakenings into sleep. In addition to bouncing back and forth between wake and sleep over the entire 24-hour period, the person with narcolepsy may also experience characteristics of REM sleep at unpredictable times.

As explained in Chapter 2, REM sleep has two unique components. One is that your mind is very active and you do most of your dreaming during REM sleep. The other is that your body becomes "paralyzed," undergoing a complete loss of voluntary muscle tone. This keeps your body from acting out your dreams.

A person with narcolepsy is prone to having one or the other of these conditions occur at the wrong times, during his or her waking life, during the onset of sleep, or during the period of waking up.

The most dramatic example of such occurrences is a state called cataplexy, in which a conscious, alert individual can lose muscle tone and suffer partial or total collapse. When the cataplexy, which literally means "to strike down with fear," affects the major muscles of the body, this sudden collapse looks like a hit from a stun gun.

Sixty to 80 percent of people with narcolepsy suffer from cataplexy. It can be triggered by surprise, fear, anger, or laughter. It also occurs more frequently during times of stress or fatigue. The effects include slight feelings of weakness and sagging facial muscles, head nodding, buckling knees, loss of arm strength, and mumbling or "garbled" speech. But it may also lead to immediate total body collapse; a person may appear unconscious to onlookers, but remain awake and alert. These attacks may last from a few seconds to half an hour or so. There is no loss of consciousness. When muscle control returns, the person is entirely awake and alert.

According to recent research, cataplexy results in part from sudden reductions in the levels of the neurotransmitter norepinephrine, which helps maintain muscle tone. Norepinephrine is very similar to epinephrine, which is also known as adrenaline. Both neurotransmitters are chemical messengers for the sympathetic nervous system, which not only helps the body maintain its normal muscle tone but helps respond to short-term stress—fight or flight, as we called it in Chapters 6 and 10. Remember what happens during an episode of sleep apnea? The body responds to a blockage of the airway by sending out a chemical jolt. That is the sympathetic nervous system at work.

Norepinephrine also helps maintain the flow of blood that keeps your muscles functioning normally. At night when you're asleep, you don't need the same degree of muscle tone because you aren't using your arms and legs. But you need it during the day. If the secretion of norepinephrine cuts out during the day in response to excitement of one kind or another, you lose control of these muscles. That's what happens during cataplexy. A decrease in serotonin may also be involved in the cataplexy response. At the same time, levels of histamine, which is now thought to control wakefulness, are unaltered. As you will read, however, most of the current thinking on narcolepsy/cataplexy centers on brain proteins called orexins.

The Babysitter Needed a Babysitter

Ellen, a nursing student, made extra money by babysitting for a family member. She had to find a new line of casual labor, however, when she almost dropped a baby in her care because she suffered an episode of narcolepsy while burping the child.

With treatment, combining a series of strategically timed naps and a drug called Provigil, she completed her studies and has found a successful niche in an area of nursing practice that can accommodate her condition.

A Tetrad of Symptoms

Excessive daytime sleepiness and cataplexy are two of a group of four—what we call a *tetrad*—symptoms that taken together make for a definitive diagnosis of narcoplepsy. The others are hypnagogic hallucinations and sleep paralysis.

Hypnagogic hallucinations are intense, convincing, and frequently frightening auditory, visual, or sensory perceptions that occur at times that have nothing to do with normal sleep—usually at the onset of sleep, which for people with narcolepsy is a frequent event during the day. This is the special effects REM counterpart of cataplexy; instead of paralysis, there is malfunction of the dream component of REM sleep.

The visual hallucinations have been compared to a video or film running in the head or a waking dream with strong emotional content, which can be pretty disturbing, as all emotional dreams can be. They may, however, also take the form of visions of colored forms that change sizes and shapes. Hypnagogic hallucinations can also occur among people without narcolepsy, although they are usually less vivid and more fragmentary than with narcolepsy.

Auditory hallucinations range from random sounds to full melodies. And physical hallucinations range from the sensation of rubbing or light touching to levitation.

I find that narcoleptic patients are less willing to talk about these hallucinations than other symptoms. Some who have them profess not to recognize that there's anything abnormal going on because they are so used to them. Those who have these hallucinations are often so embarrassed over "spacing out" in this fashion that they have never spoken to anyone about them prior to seeking treatment. Or they are embarrassed by the very personal content, which is as subject to the mysterious workings of the unconscious as any dream. Or they may be worried about incipient mental illness.

These episodes may also cause great anxiety, and once they are explained clinically there's almost palpable relief. Some people are shocked to hear that this is something associated with narcolepsy, as opposed to, say, schizophrenia. They sit there slowly shaking their heads in affirmation as you describe the typical event as if they are watching one of their own personal "videos" being played back.

Sleep paralysis, another of the four symptoms, is a temporary inability to move. However, unlike cataplexy, it doesn't occur during the active part of the day. Rather, it happens while the person is in bed falling asleep or waking up, while the brain is partially sleeping and partially awake. This again can be understood as a faulty switch regulating the transition from sleeping and waking states. The mind is conscious or nearly so, but the body is unable to move.

Unlike cataplexy, sleep paralysis is not triggered by emotion. The paralysis usually lasts longer than the shortest cataplexy attacks. It can also be accompanied by vivid hallucinations. This combination of paralysis and hallucinations can be frightening, especially if it follows daytime sleepiness as the first additional symptom of narcolepsy, when the individual is unaware of any problem.

Sleep paralysis by itself is not rare. It is not necessarily a symptom of active or incipient narcolepsy. It occurs in 2–6 percent of the general population. I have several patients with a genetic form of sleep paralysis, which appears not to be related to narcolepsy.

In some cases where the symptom appears, a detailed family history may uncover an older relative who had similar symptoms in the days before we understood these states as we do now. It is something that many people have traditionally chosen to live with.

However, in light of what we know about narcolepsy, this condition is worth exploring medically, particularly if the symptoms are frightening. If the medical interview, physical examination, and final evaluation reveal no other concerns, no further testing is needed. Such patients are usually relieved to hear that the condition is fairly common and harmless. I do, however, recommend follow-up.

Associated symptoms

In addition to the tetrad of symptoms mentioned above, there are associated symptoms, including severely fragmented or disturbed sleep and automatic behavior.

Some patients have what are called "microsleeps." They behave automatically without being aware of their actions. Neither the patients nor the people around them initially recognize the behavior as part of a disorder. Rather, it may be seen as eccentricity, a symptom of stress, or the result of preoccupation with pressing concerns. Examples include:

- Driving or walking competently but ending up in the wrong place
- Jumping from one topic to another during a conversation, or just fading out and saying nothing at all
- Bizarre actions, such as putting clothing in the refrigerator
- Severe forgetfulness
- Suddenly going into slow motion and clumsiness
- Behavior that mimics certain forms of epilepsy

As time wears on, however, these symptoms of undiagnosed narcolepsy become harder to ignore. Changes in your own perception of how you feel and in the way others treat you can give rise to depression. As you are treated for depression, you may have side effects from medication. Leading a normal life becomes harder and harder.

Hard to Diagnose, Hard to Identify With

Even though narcolepsy is fairly common, it is underdiagnosed. The best estimates are that only 25 percent of actual cases are currently diagnosed. Part of the problem is that people who begin to exhibit symptoms try to treat themselves by changing their sleep routine, drinking more coffee, surrendering to the impulse to nap, and so forth.

A teacher at a local junior high—not the teacher I mentioned in the Introduction—used to assign classwork and then put her head down on her desk while the students worked. She was narcoleptic and suffering from excessive daytime sleepiness. It was years before she sought medical treatment, and even then, her doctors ran many tests for other conditions before they would refer her to a sleep clinic. In the past, narcolepsy was not high on the list of conditions suspected to cause pathologic daytime sleepiness. However, for most GPs or other specialists it is now moving rapidly up into the top 10.

Narcolepsy on the Job

The case of Margaret is typical of the confusion and disruption that untreated narcolepsy can engender in the life of a typical worker. Fourteen years ago, this 47-year-old female travel agent consulted me, complaining of insomnia. Margaret had a history of substance abuse and eating disorders. She smoked cigarettes and drank. With a full menu of sleep-disrupting factors like that to wade through, I didn't immediately suspect narcolepsy. There were many other behavioral reasons why her sleep would suffer.

As we were discussing her history, Margaret happened to mention, "One day when I was talking to a customer who had missed a flight, I couldn't put three words together. The customer started yelling at me, 'Are you an idiot? What are you talking about? I'm stuck at the airport and you're talking nonsense.'"

This anecdote suggested to me that narcolepsy might be involved, and I began to ask her a different set of questions. What unfolded was an account of a lifetime of misery. She had an incredible secret history: sleepiness as a child, poor grades, demoralization, shame, depression, social isolation; fear of sleep because of sleep paralysis, waking nightmares in living color, lost job opportunities; and years of searching for substances to fill the void left by the random drifting between the world of sleep and waking.

Because of her history of substance abuse, she was initially reluctant to take any medication under my care. Fortunately, since the attacks of severe sleepiness were infrequent and her cataplexy was mild, we were able to structure an initial treatment plan that included scheduled naps, minimal medication, and improved sleep hygiene. After overcoming her well-founded fears about substance abuse, we tried almost every medication possible.

By reaching out to others with narcolepsy, she gained insight into her condition, with the added perk of finding support and timely information updates via the Internet.

Now, with the newfound knowledge of her condition and the cooperation and understanding of her sympathetic employers as well as a disciplined medication regimen, she has been able to continue to work productively.

As usually happens in treating people with narcolepsy, the battle to get her back to a more earth-friendly existence was a long one. Counseling and support groups helped her gain a deeper understanding of her illness. Knowledge and the process of sharing information were themselves therapeutic. With a combination of treatments helping her deal with her narcolepsy, she is now living a healthier and happier life.

Narcolepsy—The Cost in Quality of Life

You will recall from the Introduction the despair of a dedicated teacher whose narcolepsy was so debilitating that she sought treatment with an experimental drug in spite of severe potential side effects. This is very common. In fact, in a study of quality of life impact of three disabling diseases—Parkinson's disease, epilepsy, and narcolepsy—people with narcolepsy fared very poorly. Subjects were measured according to eight criteria: physical function, physical role limitations, body pain, general health, vitality, social function, emotional role limitations, and mental health.

Narcolepsy patients fared no better than people with the other two conditions on any measure, and came in last on both vitality and social function. Why does narcolepsy hit its victims so hard?

A big part of it is age of onset. Symptoms of Parkinson's typically don't appear until the age of 60, which means that patients have enjoyed most of their lives without it. But people with narcolepsy, who are usually afflicted by the age of 25, have to live with their condition through what should be their formative and most productive years. It hurts their performance in school and at work and limits their earning capacity. It makes it harder to make friends and lovers, and thus start families of their own. They have more accidents than the general population, but the discomfort they feel from their medicine prompts many to choose between medication and safety. In some countries, they are not allowed to drive at all.

To put it concisely, narcolepsy keeps people from becoming the people they might have been.

Poor Reception

Narcoleptic symptoms are embarrassing, too. People are marked by the spectacle of nodding off at a dinner party or collapsing in the middle of a burst of laughter. This behavior is imputed to lack of self-control, drinking, and substance abuse. The entertainer Liz Winstead, formely of Air America Radio, recalled on the air how for years before she was diagnosed with narcolepsy, her friends used to think that she just couldn't hold her liquor. To imagine the stigma attached to narcolepsy, consider the following, which I found after an Internet search using the keywords "narcolepsy" and "celebrities." I found an entry from June 3, 2003, about an actress whose dog was rushed to the hospital. A tabloid reported that the dog had swallowed a bag of marijuana when in fact the dog had a form of narcolepsy.

Dogs suffer from narcolepsy, caused, apparently, by mutated receptor genes in the brain, which produce receptor cells for substances called orexins that help regulate sleep and wakefulness. The most telling symptom is cataplexy, and like human attacks, they are provoked by excitement, such as feeding or play.

With humans, the problem seems to lie not with the receptor cells themselves but with the cells that make the orexins. Still, while the causes of human and canine narcolepsy may be different, studies of animal behavior are yielding important information for diagnosis and possible treatment in human beings.

What Causes Narcolepsy?

The current thinking is that an important group of cells in the brain responsible for sleep-wake behavior is damaged or absent. The small grouping of cells in the hypothalamus produce the neuroproteins called orexin, referred to earlier, or hypocretin, a neurotransmitter known to be involved in not only the sleep-wake arousal system but also in muscle movement, metabolism, heart rate, and blood pressure control. The spinal fluid of most patients with narcolepsy shows this neuroprotein lacking or deficient. Many animals with narcolepsy show a similar deficiency in orexins.

Abnormalities in orexins can result from genetics or direct damage to the hypothalamus. One continuing area for study is the association of narcolepsy and a gene that codes for a genetic marker called HLA, or human leukocyte antigen (white blood cell molecule), which can be measured in the blood. The HLA marker is also associated with other autoimmune conditions such as multiple sclerosis, some forms of arthritis, and diabetes.

How this genetic tendency is related to the orexin protein and pathway remains to be determined. There may be some connection to environmental factors. Infection, direct damage to the hypothalamus, and autoimmune disease, where the body's defensive systems turn on the body itself, disturbing the orexin cells, may contribute to narcolepsy. Recent research has correlated narcolepsy with birth month. The linkage is thought to be based on seasonal illness of the mother during a critical period of pregnancy, when the hypothalamus is developing.

There are two types of narcolepsy, "familial," which means that it runs in families, and the move common "sporadic" narcolepsy representing 95 percent of cases. In my practice, I have a three-generation family with narcolepsy. The grandmother had all the symptoms but was not diagnosed. My patient has full-blown, severe narcolepsy. There are three daughters, two of whom have narcolepsy, and a son with multiple sclerosis.

While there may be no neat hereditary line of narcolepsy between one generation and another, if you have narcolepsy, the risk of narcolepsy for "first-degree" relatives, such as brothers, sisters or children, is much higher (a 1–2 percent risk, compared with .05 percent risk for the population at large).

Diagnosing Narcolepsy

While excessive daytime sleepiness (EDS) is usually the first symptom, and for some, the *only* symptom of early narcolepsy, it is also a symptom of various other medical conditions. As I said earlier, a decade or more may elapse between the onset of narcolepsy symptoms and a definitive diagnosis. In the meantime, the patient may suffer through stages such as denial and self-medication, followed by misdiagnosis for depression, chronic fatigue syndrome, and many other disorders.

Cataplexy, which is almost unique to narcolepsy, makes the diagnosis much easier. (To see examples of cataplexy, go to the Stanford University Web site: www.med.standford.edu/school/psychiatry/narcolepsy and click on "movie-cataplexy.")

In most cases, laboratory tests are still needed to confirm diagnosis and determine a treatment plan. The usual procedure includes an overnight polysomnogram (PSG) at a sleep disorders center to look for other causes of EDS and to assess narcolepsy sleep physiology. When added to a good history the multiple sleep latency test (MSLT) is the clincher—during nap opportunities people with narcolepsy fall asleep an average of 6 minutes after their heads hit the pillow, compared with 19 minutes for normal sleepers. (For a description of the MSLT, see Chapter 4.) HLA blood testing, as discussed, is not a definitive test but it can help in the event of a questionable diagnosis, and perhaps add to our collective knowledge. Research on the orexin protein discussed earlier may lead to new and more accurate tests and treatment options for narcolepsy.

Treating Narcolepsy

The first step to treatment is to understand the condition. When I talk with a patient newly diagnosed with narcolepsy, I usually hear these questions: "How did I get it?" "Will I have it my whole life?" "Can my children get it from me?" By now you have answers to these questions. Treatment, however, involves understanding, coupled with disciplined management. The working world is not sympathetic to people with severe symptoms of narcolepsy. Society expects us to be awake during the working day and is generally intolerant of those whose bodies tell them to sleep. Still, if you have a mild case of this condition and understand it well enough to shape your behavior and educate your employers sufficiently, it can be managed. The fit is not perfect, any more than being dyslexic or, say, driving an American car on English roads, but with the right level of commitment, discipline, and medication if necessary, you can lead a satisfying and productive life. Since we don't have the magic bullet to fix narcolepsy yet, we must manage symptoms and optimize our 24-hour day. As in any other sleep disorder, this means correcting nighttime or sleep problems as well as the disruptive daytime symptoms.

Narcolepsy Treatment

Understanding How Narcolepsy Affects You

Controlling Symptoms

A. Excessive Daytime Sleepiness (EDS)

	Drug name	Description
Stimulant Drug Therapy	Modafinil (Provigil)	Mechanism of action not known
	Methylphenidate (Ritalin)	Amphetamine-like
	Dextroamphetamine (Dexedrine)	Amphetamine
	Methamphetamine (Desoxyn)	Amphetamine
	Pemoline (Cylert)	

B. Cataplexy and Other REM Symptoms

	Drug name	Description
REM Suppressing Drugs	Venlafaxine (Effexor)	Unique action
	Atomoxetine (Strattera)	Norepinephrine enhancers
	Protriptyline (Vivactil)	Tricyclic antidepressants
	Clomipramine (Anafranil)	
	Imipramine (Elavil)	
	Selegiline (Eldepryl)	Monoamine oxidase inhibitor
	Paroxetine (Paxil)	Selective serotonin reuptake inhibitors
	Sertraline (Zoloft)	
	Fluoxetine (Prozac)	
	Reboxetine (Edronex)	Noradrenaline reuptake inhibitor

C. EDS, Cataplexy, and Poor Nighttime Sleep
Combine A or B above with sleeping pill, i.e., hypnotic
Sodium Oxybate (Xyrem)

Nondrug Therapy for All Symptoms

Forced naps, good sleep hygiene, avoiding sedating medications and alcohol, caution combining other meds, regular doctor visits, realistic work-rest schedule, avoiding shift work, creating support systems

Life Management Strategies

"PEP" = Participate, Educate, and Propagate information to employers, teachers, family, friends about narcolepsy

Join support groups

Address legal, disability, and safety issues

Make the most of your individual "power hours" every day

Disclaimer: The contents of this chart, *and of this book,* are for information only and should not be used as a substitute for a doctor visit. This is a partial list and symptoms or treatment should be discussed with your doctor.

Given our current state of knowledge, most people with narcolepsy can optimize their 24-hour day through a combination of medications designed to override the faulty switch that regulates waking, sleep, and REM sleep, together with a planned "catch it while you can" sleep schedule. Thomas Edison practiced a form of narcolepsy in reverse by napping on his lab couch with both arms dangling to the side and holding palm-sized steel balls. When he entered deep sleep, or REM sleep, his hands would relax and the noise from the bouncing balls would awaken him enough so that he could peer into the dream state and get what he called "dream insight." This helped him solve the problem of the day. He was using muscle paralysis to signal REM sleep and then trying to intrude the reasoning and recall of wakefulness into the dream state. If you have narcolepsy, you will recognize this process in the other direction. Unwanted REM physiology causes muscle weakness in the form of cataplexy, or sleep attacks, and this intrudes into your wake state.

Treatment of narcolepsy is constantly changing based on new research describing the causes. Accordingly we combine new treatment with the old standbys, which include medication, behavioral therapy such as forced naps, and good sleep hygiene.

Drug Treatments
STIMULANTS

Benefits include improved mood, mental acuity, and other mental functioning.

Common side effects include weight loss, dizziness, nausea, changes in blood pressure, rapid heartbeat, and headache.

People with heart disease, hyperthyroidism, glaucoma, anxiety disorder, and high blood pressure should avoid stimulants or take them only under a physician's guidance.

These stimulants are standard treatments for narcolepsy:

Modafinil

The closest we have to a breakthrough in the safe treatment of the daytime sleepiness of narcolepsy is modafinil, sold as Provigil and Alertec, which promotes long-lasting wakefulness. Before treatment, patients in one study were able to stay awake only an average of 6 minutes out of 20 in a multiple sleep latency test (MSLT). After treatment, their waking increased to 12 to 14 minutes and some had normal wake times. Another study showed that modafinil increased the ability to stay awake by 50 percent and reduced involuntary sleep episodes by about 25 percent.

Modafinil has numerous other benefits. For example, it doesn't appear to have any harmful effects when taken with Ritalin. Furthermore, people who use it do not build up a tolerance. It does not appear to interfere with the natural hormones that play a big role in sleep, including cortisol (the major stress hormone), melatonin, and growth hormone. Therefore, studies show no interference with voluntary daytime or with nighttime sleep.

In addition, modafinil seems to cause less anxiety than standard stimulants. It also seems to have less potential for abuse than other stimulants. There's no "rebound effect"—the crushing depression, disorientation, and lethargy that amphetamine users experience when their drugs wear off and they "crash." One trial showed no signs of addiction or habituation after up to nine weeks of daily use.

Insurance companies have often been reluctant to pay for Provigil, which costs nearly $300 per month, preferring that doctors prescribe the cheaper Ritalin, even for patients with high blood pressure, which is a known side effect. This and other treatment battles can be fought and won. There are also problems with the level of dosage. Insurance companies have frequently been willing to reimburse only for prescription at a 200-milligram dose, which may well be too high for some people. One person's maintenance dose of any stimulant may be another person's multiday burst of speed. Modafinil is less prone to such complications than other stimulants, but it does have its share of problems. Versions of the drug now under development promise to be more effective still. As the patents for the first generation of modafinil expire and generic versions become available, finely targeted dosages will become easier to prescribe.

In addition modafinil is now being used to treat other causes of daytime sleepiness and it was found to be safe for use in children with disorders such as ADHD. Promising as it is, however, modafinil does not work for every case of narcolepsy.

Side effects include the following:

- Headache (the most commonly reported side effect)
- Nausea
- Diarrhea
- Dry mouth
- Nasal and throat congestion

- Nervousness
- Dizziness

Modafinil may also interfere with the effectiveness of birth control pills. Women of childbearing age who take modafinil should switch to other methods of birth control. Recently cases of valvular heart disease have been reported. If there is a concern based on your history or physical examination, an echocardiogram may be required prior to the start of the medication. Discuss this with your doctor.

It should be noted that patients who are switching from another agent to modafinil must discuss the process carefully with their physicians. Withdrawal symptoms from stimulants while switching over may be particularly difficult, and may include the return of symptoms such as EDS.

During withdrawal, patients should avoid driving!

Methylphenidate (Ritalin, Ritalin-SR), 10–100 Mg

This is currently one of the most frequently prescribed stimulants for treatment of narcolepsy in the United States. It is less potent than dextroamphetamine or methamphetamine. It is available in a regular or long-acting form, SR (sustained release). It can be used in combination with some other stimulants. It is a Schedule II medication in the United States, which means that quantities and refills are strictly controlled by government regulation.

Side effects include mood changes and muscle tremors. It should not be used during pregnancy. There is the risk of psychosis, depression, overdose, addiction, and abuse.

Dextroamphetamine, Dextroamphetamine-Sulfate (DexedrineR, Dextro-Stat, Dexedrine-SR), 5–100 Mg

It also comes in a regular and prolonged-action form, SR (sustained release). It is also strictly controlled and is a Schedule II medication.

Methamphetamine-HCI (Desoxyn), 5–100 Mg

This is more potent than the previous two dextroamphetamines, but otherwise similar in action.

Pemoline (Cylert), 37.5–300 Mg

Less potent than other stimulants, this is a Schedule IV medication in the United States, so prescriptions can be refilled for up to six months without seeing a doctor each time. It can cause liver damage, however, and is not commonly used at this time.

Tip for Using Stimulants: Take a Day Off

As with most mood-altering drugs, your body develops a tolerance to these drugs. That is, they become less effective if used every day, leaving you with the choice of taking continually larger doses or trying to control your dependence on them. Patients are advised to take "drug holidays" one day per week or to withdraw gradually and resume treatment at a lower dosage, and by all means, work closely with your doctor.

REM SUPPRESSING DRUGS FOR CATAPLEXY AND OTHER REM SYMPTOMS

Antidepressants are used to control abnormal REM. For example, antidepressants have been shown to be very effective in controlling symptoms of cataplexy.

Monoamine Oxidase Inhibitors (Selegiline)

Selegiline (Eldepryl), also known as **deprenyl,** is an **antioxidant** drug that blocks **monoamine oxidase B,** an enzyme that degrades dopamine and may contribute to narcolepsy. Selegiline has side effects, such as adverse interactions with most antidepressants, some very serious. People taking monoamine oxidase inhibitors are at risk for high blood pressure if they consume tyramine-containing foods or beverages, including aged cheeses, most red wines, vermouth, dried meats and fish, canned figs, fava beans, and concentrated yeast products.

The tricyclic antidepressants **protriptyline (Vivactil), clomipramine (Anafranil), imipramine (Janimine, Tofranil),** and **viloxazine (Vivalan),** appear to suppress REM sleep and may be used in conjunction with stimulants in severe cases.

These antidepressants do not cause unusual drowsiness and are useful for managing cataplexy, sleep paralysis, and hypnagogic hallucinations. However, the common side effects of these medications make them intolerable to many patients. The most often reported include the following:

- Dry mouth
- Constipation
- Blurred vision
- Sexual dysfunction
- Weight gain
- Difficulty in urinating
- Drowsiness
- Dizziness (Blood pressure may drop suddenly when sitting up or standing.)

Tricyclics can have serious, although rare, side effects, such as disturbances in heart rhythm and their possible connection to a lung disease called idiopathic pulmonary fibrosis (IPF), which can cause lung inflammation and scarring. Initial symptoms are breathlessness and dry cough.

Overdoses can be fatal.

Selective Serotonin Reuptake Inhibitors (SSRIs)

These antidepressants may also be helpful in combination with stimulants. For example, venlafaxine (Effexor) which also blocks reuptake of norepinephrine and serotonin, fluoxetine (Prozac, the standard SSRI), and citalopram (Celexa), another SSRI, have been reported to be effective in treating cataplexy that does not respond to standard treatments. Side effects include the following:

- Nausea and gastrointestinal problems, which usually wear off over time
- Dry mouth and increased risk of cavities and mouth sores
- Headache
- Some weight loss during the first few weeks of treatment, but patients typically return to their pretreatment weight
- Sexual dysfunction, including delayed orgasm or loss of orgasm and low sexual drive, occurs in 30–40 percent of patients on SSRIs. (Citalopram may pose a lower risk for this side effect than other SSRIs.)

Agitation, insomnia, mild tremor, and impulsivity occur in 10–20 percent of people who take SSRIs, which may be problematic in patients who also suffer from anxiety, sleeplessness, or both. Such side effects may persist. On the other hand, about 20 percent of SSRI-treated patients experience drowsiness, which can be useful if the medication is taken at bedtime.

Other Antidepressants

Certain drugs, which are also known as "designer" drugs, are targeted at a very narrow set of neuropathways. They are likely to be more common in the future. Reboxetine (Edronex) is a unique antidepressant, known as a selective noradrenaline reuptake inhibitor and has shown some efficacy in reducing daytime sleepiness.

A DRUG THAT DECREASES REM SYMPTOMS AND IMPROVES SLEEP AND DAYTIME ALERTNESS

Combinations of medications can be used to treat multiple symptoms. There are limitations to this method, however, including side effects, drug interactions, and difficulty in keeping to an elaborate drug regimen.

There is one medication that treats almost all the symptoms of narcolepsy: sodium oxybate, which is sold under the brand name Xyrem. It is taken only at bedtime with an additional dose three to four hours later. It appears to improve healthy sleep, relieve daytime sleepiness, and control cataplexy. But while it has been approved by the FDA, it is also an extreme example of what a mixed blessing pharmaceuticals can be. A form of this drug called gamma-hydroxybutyrate (GHB) has achieved notoriety as the "date rape drug" and has been sold as a street drug under the names "Grievous Bodily Harm" or "Liquid Ecstasy." Very serious side effects, including seizures, coma, and respiratory arrest, have been reported. Xyrem is only available through a centralized pharmacy and is closely monitored because of the potential for abuse and serious side effects.

Sodium oxybate is a central nervous system depressant and should be taken only immediately prior to sleep as it is listed as a strong hypnotic sedative. It may cause drowsiness if taken during the day and you should not drive, operate machinery, or perform other hazardous activities for at least six hours after taking it. In fact, such activities should be avoided altogether while taking the medication. There may be serious interactions with other medications, antihistamines, sedatives (used to treat insomnia), seizure medicines, and muscle relaxants, to name a few. *Never* take any other medicine while under treatment with sodium oxybate without first talking to your doctor.

Sodium oxybate is habit-forming and you can become physically and psychologically dependent on it. Withdrawal symptoms may occur, so any attempt to curtail its use should be done under the supervision of your doctor, who may recommend a gradual reduction in dosage.

There are many other precautions listed for sodium oxybate including warnings not to take the medication if you have other medical conditions, a history of psychiatric disorders, or if you are pregnant, breast feeding, or over 65.

Side effects include:

- Allergic reaction, such as difficulty breathing; closing of the throat; swelling of the lips, face, or tongue; hives; hallucinations or severe confusion
- Sleepwalking

Other, less serious side effects may be more likely to occur:

- Drowsiness
- Dizziness
- Headache
- Nausea, vomiting, diarrhea, or abdominal pain
- Weakness
- Depression
- Urinary or fecal incontinence
- Nervousness
- Increased sweating
- Abnormal dreams

(Source: Adapted from Cerner Multum, Inc. Version: 1.03. Revision date: 2/13/04.)

INVESTIGATIVE DRUGS

Other drugs that might be beneficial under certain circumstances are the antiseizure drug carbamazepine (Tegretol) and the opiate codeine. These drugs can cause among other things orthostatic hypotension, an abrupt drop in blood pressure after standing up.

Early experiments with the protein hypocretin, or orexin, are showing significant results in treatments of narcoleptic dogs, including dramatic improvement in cataplexy, duration of waking time, and the ability to remain asleep.

Nondrug Treatments

For narcolepsy, as for other sleep disorders, or indeed most medical problems of any kind, the best treatment has a strong element of behavioral change. We must let the body treat itself whenever we can.

Behavioral treatment for narcolepsy calls for three or more scheduled naps throughout the day. One study calls for combining scheduled nighttime sleep with two 15-minute naps, one before lunch and another before dinner. Patients should also steer clear of heavy meals and alcohol, both of which can interfere with sleep even for nonnarcoleptics.

How effective are naps for people on stimulants to treat narcolepsy? Do they add any benefit? Does the combination of medication and napping "cure" narcolepsy? The answer is not the same for everyone. Those who can remain alert while on medication or who are only moderately sleepy generally derive no additional benefit from naps. For those who are still extremely sleepy in spite of medication, however, naps are necessary.

Even if stimulants seem to do the trick, continual care should be a fact of life. Just as people on Lipitor or other cholesterol-lowering drugs shouldn't use it as a license to eat beef three times a day, so people with narcolepsy must manage their medication with care.

Alternative and "Natural" Remedies

People with chronic medical problems that resist "cure" with standard medical treatment are constantly on the lookout for miracles. No one can blame them. They crave normality. Being on your guard against the illness all the time is frustrating; it limits your enjoyment of pleasures most people take for granted; and it's expensive to boot.

It's this combination of factors that leaves many people with arthritis, chronic pain, asthma, allergies, acne, high blood pressure, and many other conditions open to quackery—usually abetted by a fair dose of conspiracy theories about the monopoly of traditional medicine.

I assure you, however, that there's no vast medical conspiracy at work when it comes to narcolepsy. As described earlier, the best medical evidence points in the direction of deficient production of certain neurotransmitters for which there currently is no cure. For now, the best way to control the effects of this problem is to sleep strategically and if necessary augment this with a lot of acceptance and the least amount of effective chemistry.

The designation "alternative" or "natural" when used in conjunction with such medication doesn't mean that it's more in tune with some version of God's plan than the most refined laboratory creation. Don't forget, many, many patented drugs from aspirin to Taxol (a treatment for breast cancer) began with some plant somewhere. Instead of searching the Internet for a miracle cure, you should go to a sleep specialist and spend your spare time supporting efforts to preserve the rain forests. If the rain forests survive, it's more likely that some competent scientist will find a cure for your narcolepsy some day than that you will ever be cured by some current alternative narcolepsy treatment. The eventual cure, however, is more likely to come from a fix in the genetic instruction for the proteins controlling or involved in the hypocretin pathway or with a drug that does the job of hypocretin.

If alternative or natural remedies have any effect at all, it's because they contain some powerful chemical. A case in point for narcolepsy is ephedrine, a derivative of the herb *ma huang* (ephedra). This stimulant, once used in ancient China to keep guards awake, has now been banned from over-the-counter preparations after a baseball player died while using it to lose weight. Side effects are the same as with prescription stimulants, including insomnia, motor disturbances, high blood pressure, glaucoma, impaired cerebral circulation, urinary disturbances, and unstable blood sugar levels.

These preparations are unregulated. Their quality is not controlled nor their effectiveness proved. There have been a number of reported cases of serious and even lethal side effects from herbal products. In spite of the designation "natural," they might be as close to nature as the gasoline in your car is to the crude oil that was used to manufacture it. Some have even been found to contain standard prescription medications.

For more information on natural remedy brands log on to http://www.ConsumerLab.com. The Food and Drug Administration has a program called MEDWATCH that enables people to report adverse reactions to untested substances, such as herbal remedies and vitamins (call 800-332-1088).

Managing Life with Narcolepsy

The goal in treating narcolepsy is to bypass the faulty switch that regulates the states of waking and sleep as much as possible, or at least create and control your schedule of sleep with forced and timed scheduled naps and medication. Your journey through space and time can be as productive as that of those without narcolepsy. After all, it's your journey.

Some of the ways to manage narcolepsy include the following:

- Learn as much as you can about narcolepsy and your symptoms. Keep a log of your activities to help you figure out events and behavior that bring on cataplexy, which should help you change your routine to better manage your symptoms and avoid injury.
- Talk with your doctor often. Keep her or him informed about your symptoms and about your daily life, as well as any side effects you may be having from medications you are taking.
- Join a support group of individuals who are going through the same things you are. You can learn a lot about how others cope with similar symptoms and get emotional support, but avoid groups that promise quick cures. If something sounds too good to be true, it probably is, as the saying goes.
- Build a support system, not just a support group, but one that includes family, friends, employer, and teachers as well—anyone you trust or must rely on in the course of your routine. Talk with them about your condition and work out what they can do to help you manage it. Above all, this will persuade them that you are not lazy, hostile, unmotivated, or bored—all common assumptions others make about people with narcolepsy. Try to persuade employers or teachers to work with you to devise an appropriate schedule.
- In addition to regular nap times, exercise and make sure you get enough sleep (around eight hours) every night.
- Talk to a counselor or mental health provider experienced with working with people with disabilities. Such counseling should help you to cope with personal, family, and work-related issues.

You should not be employed at any job requiring long drives or the operation of hazardous equipment or materials, or that requires prolonged alertness without a break.

As with many other disorders, narcolepsy has a profound impact not only on those with the condition but those around them. Considering the relatively short time since the discovery of REM and our ever-improving understanding of the genetic and neurological pathways involved, we look forward to a cure in the near future. Meanwhile, we must protect the person with narcolepsy not only from injury but from the personal misery and isolation that their condition can bring.

Kindred Spirit

While it will be years before there is a cure for narcolepsy, the frontiers of treatment will probably depend as much on patients themselves as on doctors and scientists. This is because as in many other fields of medicine, networks of patients are often more effective at getting the word out about current developments than are their doctors.

One such person is Audrey Kindred, a patient of mine, who is a member of the board of Narcolepsy Network. She is now an active community leader, advocate, and teacher. In a recent newsletter, she described how "narcolepsy had wreaked its havoc and confusion upon my life, and I faced an anger that felt foreign and overwhelming to me. My identity as a person with narcolepsy was acute at this point, red and hot and sore in me like a wound. Diagnosis had revealed to me the name of my nemesis: Narcolepsy. One name for the endless blurry experiences in which I'd been floating for years."

Audrey now helps organize conferences for the Network, something her friends find highly amusing as they imagine a "room of bobbing heads." For Audrey, "Learning and shedding light upon the mysterious experiences of narcolepsy is a core motivation for me in both creating and attending these conferences. Implicitly it is among my life's missions to explore the very particular angle on life with which I am endowed. Likewise, you are each experts of your own experience.

"Yet, too often we are isolated, unrepresented, and perhaps even uncertain of our relevance to the awake world. In the conference experience, I see us all as personal researchers comparing heart-felt notes on the far inner reaches of our experience, finding company and recognition and relevance for our narcoleptic uniqueness and mutually cultivating the tools for our growth. There is so much for us to learn and explore as a community. . . . Narcolepsy consciousness in this decade is awakening. As we wake up, let us also dream ever more."

9

RESTLESS LEGS—PAIN IN MOTION

When I lecture on limb movement disorders, in which sleep is disturbed or interrupted by pain and movement, I start with the case of a patient at our lab. At intervals throughout the night he would reach down and punch his lower legs five or six times then go back to sleep. We later found out that his bedtime routine included positioning a piece of wood the size of a small baseball bat next to his bed for easy access to bang away at his legs. Although we do tell patients to "bring along anything that is part of your bedtime routine" to help them feel comfortable in the sleep lab bedroom, he felt awkward bringing his Louisville Slugger. The night at the lab without his usual equipment was a particularly bad one. He described the discomfort as an intense aching, burning, and cramping in both legs that would keep him awake unless he took action.

Take the RLS Test

How do you know if you have this condition? It's so obscure that most people don't even know it exists.

1. When you sit or lie down, do you have a strong feeling or urge to move your legs that may prove impossible to resist?
2. Is this urge to move your legs associated with unpleasant or creepy-crawly sensations deep in your legs?
3. Do the sensations and urge to move tend to occur during periods of rest or inactivity?
4. Are these symptoms reduced or relieved by voluntary movement of your legs?
5. Do the sensations and urge to move bother you more in the evening and at night, especially when you lie down, than during the day?
6. Do you often have trouble falling asleep or staying asleep?
7. Does your bed partner tell you that you jerk your legs when you are asleep? Do you sometimes have involuntary leg jerks when you are awake?
8. Are you frequently tired or unable to concentrate during the day?
9. Do you have family members who experience those same urges to move and unpleasant sensations?
10. Have medical tests failed to reveal a cause for your urge to move and unpleasant sensations?

—Restless Legs Syndrome Foundation www.rls.org

Look at the language in the test above. "Unpleasant or creepy-crawly sensations deep in your legs." My patients describe bugs, worms, and fire.

Restless legs syndrome (RLS) is a neurological disorder. The nasty sensations range in severity from the merely uncomfortable to excruciating, and are accompanied by an uncontrollable urge to move, which is at its peak when you are sitting or lying still. In fact, it's relaxation and rest that set the symptoms (and the legs) in motion. Moreover, the longer people with RLS remain still, the worse their symptoms become.

You might occasionally see people in restaurants who can't sit still. They are continually moving their feet, scratching obsessively, and shifting their weight. Whether they are conscious of their movements or not doesn't matter. The important point is that they are so uncomfortable that they don't care what they look like. That guy you see pacing up and down may not be waiting for his dinner to arrive; he may merely be trying to stave off the discomfort of RLS.

Clearly, restless legs syndrome is not Steve Martin's "happy feet," a routine in which the comic's feet would spontaneously burst into dance. It's more like the movie *Alien,* in which monsters pop out of people's skin—or it feels that way.

However, as annoying as RLS can be when people are fully awake, when it is combined with sleep it becomes a much more serious problem. The symptoms are worse in the evening generally, and they are aggravated further by lying down. As you are now fully aware from having read a good deal of this book, anything that detracts from your ability to get a good night's sleep compromises your health and quality of life. According to a study in the journal *Sleep Medicine* written up in *The New York Times* (May 25, 2004), about 70 percent of chronic sufferers have problems falling asleep and 60 percent awaken at least three times a night. This causes sleep onset insomnia and sleep maintenance insomnia: They can't get to sleep and can't stay asleep.

Research has shown that people who suffer from RLS also suffer disproportionately from anxiety, depression, and tension—and the more severe the RLS symptoms are, the higher the cost in these measures of mental health.

Eighty percent of those with RLS also suffer from periodic limb movement disorder (PLMD). Their legs move in jerks and twitches at 20- or 30-second intervals through the entire night, often waking them up. Imagine how you would feel if your bed partner poked you in the leg hard enough to wake you up two or three times a minute all night. You'd be hell on wheels. You'd be exhausted all day.

Criteria for Diagnosing RLS

1. A compelling urge to move the limbs, often associated with **paresthesias** (abnormal skin sensations such as numbness, tingling, pricking, burning, or creeping on the skin that has no objective cause) or **dysesthesias** (feelings such as burning, wetness, electric shock, pins and needles, itching, creepy-crawly sensations caused by neurological malfunction)

2. Symptoms that are worse or present only during rest and are partially or temporarily relieved by activity
3. Motor restlessness as seen in activities such as floor pacing and rubbing or banging the legs
4. Nocturnal worsening of symptoms which may get better after 5 A.M. or in severe cases persist throughout the day.

Although about 85 percent of those with RLS also experience PLMD, it is not necessary for a diagnosis of RLS. Some experience symptoms in one or both of their arms as well as their legs. Most people with RLS have sleep disturbances that result in excessive daytime sleepiness and fatigue. Adapted from International Restless Legs Study Group—1995

Who Has RLS?

Lots of us—8 percent of the population, according the RLS Foundation, or twice the percentage who have sleep apnea. The exact numbers, of course, are hard to pin down because many people with symptoms do not seek medical attention. They may be afraid they will not be taken seriously. Or they may feel that their condition is one of a kind and that it doesn't even have a name, let alone established treatments. Furthermore, doctors who themselves are unfamiliar with RLS often attribute the symptoms to insomnia, stress, arthritis, muscle cramps, aging, or anxiety.

The study in the journal *Sleep Medicine* referred to above found that 65 percent of the estimated cases of RLS seek treatment for their symptoms but only 13 percent are diagnosed.

While both men and women have RLS, slightly more women seem to have it than men. And while RLS may begin as early as infancy, those who suffer worst are middle-aged or older, and its severity appears to worsen with age as symptoms become more frequent and last longer.

Hindsight, we are often reminded, is 20/20. However, with RLS it may not be all that clear. "Growing pains" in adolescence may retrospectively be attributed to early onset RLS. Likewise, the great childhood plague of attention-deficit hyperactivity disorder—characterized by an inability to sit still—could be a symptom of RLS. (For more on childhood attention deficit, see Chapter 12.)

What Causes RLS?

In most cases, the cause of RLS is idiopathic; that is, the cause is unknown. It seems to run in families in about 50 percent of cases: If your parents had RLS, there is a 30–50 percent greater chance that you will have it. When there is a family history, RLS symptoms tend to start at an earlier age and progress more slowly than with other cases.

In other cases, however, RLS appears to be related to the following factors or conditions, although researchers do not yet know if these factors actually cause RLS.

Low iron levels, or anemia. Once iron levels or anemia are treated, patients may see a reduction in symptoms.

Chronic diseases. Kidney failure, diabetes, Parkinson's disease, and peripheral neuropathy are associated with RLS. Treating the condition often provides relief from RLS.

Pregnancy. About 15 percent of pregnant women experience RLS, especially in their last trimester. In most cases, symptoms usually disappear within a month of delivery.

Medications. Antinausea drugs (prochlorperazine or metoclopramide), antiseizure drugs (phenytoin), antipsychotic drugs (haloperidol or phenothiazine derivatives), and some cold and allergy medications may aggravate symptoms.

Caffeine, alcohol, and tobacco. These "lifestyle" drugs may aggravate or trigger symptoms in patients predisposed to RLS. Studies indicate that reducing or eliminating consumption may relieve symptoms.

Diagnosis the Old-fashioned Way

As the crazy quilt of conditions associated with RLS ought to suggest, diagnosis is more a matter of good old-fashioned clinical deduction than silver-bullet laboratory science. We have no single test for RLS. Instead, the disorder is diagnosed clinically starting with a comprehensive patient history that includes patient descriptions of symptoms, current and past medical problems, family history, medications, daytime sleep patterns and sleepiness, disturbance of sleep, or daytime function.

If the history points toward RLS, the laboratory will take over with, possibly:

Blood tests to exclude anemia, decreased iron stores, diabetes, and kidney problems.

Electromyography (test that measures electrical activity within muscle fibers) and nerve conduction studies (to test the speed of impulses through a nerve pathway). These are done to measure electrical activity in muscles and nerves, while Doppler sonography (an ultrasound technique) is done to evaluate blood flow and health of blood vessels that supply the legs.

A full sleep study, consisting of a polysomnogram that records brain waves, heartbeat, and breathing during an entire night, is undertaken in some cases to rule out other sleep disorders or evaluate the severity of associated limb or leg movements and their effect on sleep.

Children Are Hard to Diagnose

An RLS diagnosis is especially difficult to make in children because the physician relies heavily on the patient's explanations of symptoms, and the symptoms can be difficult for a child to describe. As mentioned, RLS can sometimes be misdiagnosed as "growing pains," hyperactivity, or attention deficit disorder.

Beyond Movement: How Is RLS Treated?

Continual movement brings relief to those with RLS, but all that movement is tiresome. Perpetual motion doesn't work any better for restless legs than it does in physics.

Obviously, if the condition results from an underlying disorder, such as peripheral neuropathy or diabetes, treatment of that problem will relieve the symptoms of restless legs. For patients with idiopathic RLS, however, the emphasis will be on treating the symptoms.

For mild to moderate symptoms, prevention is key. As described above, cutting down or eliminating the lifestyle choices that you know are bad for you anyway—excessive caffeine, alcohol, and tobacco—may provide some relief. Certain supplements to correct deficiencies in iron, folate, and magnesium may be taken under a physician's supervision.

Better sleep patterns and regular bedtimes can reduce symptoms. For some patients whose RLS symptoms are minimized in the early morning, changing their sleep patterns for earlier waking times allows them to make more productive use of the early hours. Regular moderate exercise helps some patients sleep better, although excessive exercise can sometimes aggravate symptoms.

Hot baths, massages, heating pads, or ice packs before bedtime can relieve symptoms in some patients.

Physicians also may suggest a variety of medications to treat RLS. Generally, physicians choose from dopaminergics, which affect the nerves that rely on the neurotransmitter dopamine, benzodiazepines (central nervous system depressants), opioids, and anticonvulsants. Dopaminergic agents, largely used to treat Parkinson's disease, have been shown to reduce RLS symptoms and PLMD and are considered the initial treatment of choice. Good short-term results of treatment with levodopa plus carbidopa have been reported, although most patients eventually will develop "augmentation," meaning that symptoms are reduced at night but begin to develop earlier in the day than usual. Dopamine agonists such as pergolide mesylate, pramipexole, and ropinirole hydrochloride may be effective in some patients and are less likely to cause augmentation.

Benzodiazepines (such as clonazepam and diazepam) may be prescribed for patients who have mild or intermittent symptoms. These drugs help patients obtain a more restful sleep but they do not fully alleviate RLS symptoms and can cause daytime sleepiness. Because these depressants also may induce or aggravate sleep apnea in some cases, they should not be used in patients with apnea or any other form of sleep-disordered breathing.

For more severe symptoms, opioids such as codeine, propoxyphene, or oxycodone may be prescribed for their ability to induce relaxation and diminish pain. Side effects include dizziness, nausea, vomiting, and the risk of addiction.

Anticonvulsants such as carbamazepine and gabapentin are also useful for some patients, as they decrease the sensory disturbances— those creeping and crawling sensations. Dizziness, fatigue, and sedation are among the possible side effects.

Unfortunately, no single drug is effective for everyone with RLS. What may be helpful to one individual may actually worsen symptoms for another. In addition, medications taken regularly may lose their effect, making it necessary to change medications periodically or use combinations.

Limb and Life

RLS is a condition that affects you while you are awake. Another set of conditions that affect you while you are asleep are referred to as "limb movement disorders." However, since the legs are most commonly involved, "leg" movement is often used in place of "limb." We will use leg and limb interchangeably here, but these movements could also affect the arms.

Periodic limb movements can cause electrocortical arousal while you are asleep. The way to picture the effect of an electrocortical arousal is to think of the response you get when you try to wake a sleeping person by yelling at them or poking them in the ribs. You hear, "Huh??!!" and a second later they've gone right back to sleep. However, the continual electrical and hormonal activity of wakening due to PLMD interferes with the restful and restorative quality of your sleep. The overall effect is what we are referring to when we diagnose PLMD.

PLMD is seen equally in both men and women and occurs more commonly with advancing age. It affects only 2 percent of the population under the age of 30, 5 percent between 30 and 50, and 25 percent between 50 and 60. Approximately 40–50 percent of the population 65 or older may have PLMD.

The movements themselves are characterized by repetitive, short (up to several seconds) flexing of the muscles in the arms or legs. The movements range from a distinct fanning of the toes and flexing of the foot or hands to kicking and flailing of the arms and legs. Sometimes oral, nasal, and abdominal movements occur.

The movements generally occur throughout the night in distinct episodes or periods that last for many minutes at a time. Within one such episode they occur every 20 to 40 seconds and last from half a second to several seconds. Sometimes patients and their bed partners do not associate these episodes with a significant medical condition and therefore will not seek treatment. When the symptoms are mild, they may escape notice by the patient altogether.

Unsurprisingly, however, when the symptoms are severe, the individual is often awakened by these jerking movements, and so is the sleeping partner, with serious effects on their quality of sleep; both may have a hard time staying awake the next day.

Often PLMD occurs together with other sleep disorders including RLS, narcolepsy, sleep apnea syndrome, or REM sleep behavior disorder. When they appear in conjunction with other sleep disorders, it is often difficult to determine which condition is primarily responsible for symptoms such as daytime sleepiness.

By the Numbers

We learn about a patient's leg movements either because we look for them or find them unexpectedly during the sleep study. Sensors placed over the calf muscle record the number of leg movements per hour of sleep. This is called the Periodic Limb Movement Index. Movements are carefully counted and converted into a number that reflects how many times they occur every hour and whether or not they disturbed sleep. This average is compared against a severity index and we use this reference to help diagnose PLMD.

We also count the number of times the movement disturbs sleep by looking at the impact of the movement on the brain wave pattern on the sleep record. If the brain wave jumps from deep sleep to a lighter stage of sleep or to a wakelike pattern, we recognize the event as an electrocortical arousal.

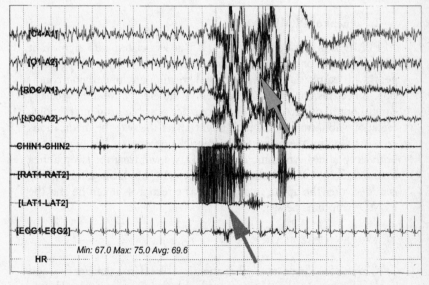

The sleep record above shows how restless leg movement can occur during sleep. The bottom arrow points to a sudden leg movement. The top arrow shows how the leg movement disrupts the sleep and causes the brain wave pattern to go from quiet sleep to a wake pattern. This represents a sudden electocortical arousal. When this happens, for example, 240 times per night, it gives an index of 40 events per hour for a six-hour sleep. This patient had exactly that index and presented to our center with severe daytime sleepiness.

To return to the poke-in-the-ribs analogy, if someone poked you 40 times an hour all night I guarantee you would be very sleepy the next day. Likewise, if the periodic limb movements come to 40 per hour with other associated symptoms, I would put it in the severe category and treatment would be warranted.

We then take the final step and try to explain the patient's presenting problem based on what we find on the sleep study. We must determine whether excessive daytime sleepiness is explained by the severity of the leg movement or if other factors are at work.

If it is determined that the limb movements are the likely cause of the symptoms and if they are severe enough, we diagnose PLMD.

This method of assigning a severity index to findings on sleep studies is very important since it helps with treatment decisions. In Chapter 6, you will recall, we used a similar concept for sleep apnea. However, charting the frequency of occurrences is just the beginning. We also ask how long did they last, and what was their effect on the brain? The answers to these questions can help us determine what to do about the problem.

Treatment of PLMD

PLMD is generally treated only if it is associated with significant RLS, insomnia, or daytime symptoms such as excessive daytime tiredness, with emphasis on reversing and treating any underlying condition. Since this condition is common in the elderly, we are especially careful not to overtreat. We must consider possible drug interactions, metabolic abnormalities, which might affect the way the medications are absorbed by the body, and potential side effects. If a person has both sleep apnea syndrome and PLMD, we will treat the sleep apnea first and then look for a clinical improvement. Medication for PLMD is added after the apnea treatment is as effective as it can be and the PLMD symptoms persist.

IRON AND THE BRAIN

We have long been aware that anemia—blood iron deficiency—and restless legs syndrome are connected, at least in some people. The relentless march of science has now shed light on a possible linkage between the way the body uses iron and RLS.

A study by James Connor, Ph.D., of Penn State College of Medicine, and others performed the first-ever autopsy analysis of the brains of people with RLS. The team examined brain tissue from seven people who had RLS, acquired through the Restless Legs Syndrome Foundation's brain collection at the Harvard Brain Bank, and five controls.

The study found that the brains of RLS subjects lacked a specific receptor for iron transport. In other words, the iron can knock on the door of the brain cells, but not all of it can come in. The brain cells are supplied with enough iron to keep them alive, but not enough to function normally. The authors hypothesize that iron deficiency may cause the neural signals to the legs to misfire, thus creating the sensations that RLS patients find so maddening.

"This doesn't necessarily mean that a person has dietary iron-deficiency and needs supplements," Dr. Connor said. "It means only that these receptors aren't packaging and delivering an adequate amount of iron to the specific cells in this portion of the brain."

There was some very good news in the study. Dr. Connor noted that "no unique pathological changes in the brains of patients with RLS" were found. "It appears that cells in a portion of the midbrain aren't getting enough iron." Unlike Parkinson's disease and Alzheimer's disease, there was no loss of brain tissue. The fact that there is no cell damage makes the prospect for successful treatment more likely.

The next order of business for this research is to isolate other potential breakdowns in the iron packaging and transport system to the brain, including genes that regulate the iron transport proteins.

"We hope these discoveries lead to a test that could diagnose this syndrome, and a potential target for a therapy to bring long-term relief to those suffering with restless legs syndrome," Connor said. More research is needed to identify the role of iron in this and other varieties of RLS.

Three Sisters

Edna had stomach surgery, and that's when her problems began. In the two years following the procedure, she began to suffer from daytime sleepiness. Her doctor diagnosed iron deficiency anemia, which is not unusual after stomach surgery, but treatment didn't solve her problems, so she came to me.

Excessive daytime sleepiness in patients with medical histories like

Edna's tends to be caused by one or more of three things—sleep apnea, poor sleep hygiene, or restless legs syndrome.

Since she also snored, we did a sleep study to rule out apnea. While her sleep hygiene wasn't the best due to the hours she kept and her nighttime eating habits, the real eye-opener was her description of leg sensations that fit the bill for RLS. She described sensations in the front of her legs as if insects were crawling under the skin, and cramping in the backs of her legs while sitting still or trying to get to sleep.

The fact that she had iron deficiency anemia made this a fairly easy diagnosis. What made the story unusual was that she had recently discovered that there was a family history of RLS.

Edna is one of three sisters. Years before, the youngest of them had gone to the hospital with complaints of EDS, which she had been experiencing for years. A sleep study showed she had periodic limb movement disorder. Like many sleep-disordered patients, she had been living with these complaints for years. Also like many others, she had tried to ignore them until they became intolerable. After her diagnosis and treatment, she told both her sisters about what had happened.

To their surprise, the other two had also been suffering with similar symptoms. That was the impetus for Edna coming to see me.

I was able to treat Edna without a sleep study. The clinical and family histories were clear enough to indicate a medication regimen. After correcting the iron deficiency, in Edna's case we used Mirapex, which is also used to treat Parkinson's—accompanied by better sleep hygiene.

Edna reflected on the story: "As the oldest sister, I had always called the shots. But maybe being the oldest also made me more willing to put up with these problems and not complain. It took my younger sister who wanted something better to show us the way."

10

INSOMNIA

When you have insomnia, you're never really asleep, and you're never really awake.

—From the movie *Fight Club,* based on the novel by Chuck Palahniuk

Unlike, say, obstructive sleep apnea, which essentially is a breathing disorder that can usually be treated by a number of physical means, insomnia is extremely complicated. Obviously the sleeping patient cannot self-report in real time, so we are left with the patient's description or interpretation of his or her own sleep—or lack of it. There are two types of insomnia: primary insomnia and secondary insomnia. Insomnia caused by another sleep disorder, another medical or psychiatric condition, the use of medication, substance abuse, or other factors that can be isolated and treated is called secondary insomnia. When insomnia exists on its own with no obvious cause, it is called primary insomnia.

Regardless of whether the condition is primary or secondary, however, the most common symptom is a preoccupation with sleeplessness. Thoughts of sleeplessness may dominate your waking days or sleepless nights. This may be more than a "mere" psychological problem, since sleeplessness has implications for our mental and physical well-being. Whichever side of the divide the insomnia originates, physical or mental, it will soon begin to affect the other, courtesy of the nervous system, which links the two. Throughout the chapter, I will refer to this model, mind and body, linked by the nervous system, as it relates to insomnia.

Evolution's Hardwiring

The human nervous system is very complex. It consists not only of both higher functions of the central nervous system, but of much more basic, involuntary brain function left over from much earlier phases of evolution.

For example, we have what is referred to now as the "enteric nervous system," which mostly has to do with the quest for food that characterizes all life-forms. Even the lowly plankton, at the bottom of the food chain, probably has some mechanism that drives it to acquire nourishment.

On top of that, we have what's called the autonomic nervous system, which is by dictionary definition "that part of the nervous system that functions more or less independently of the will." It is concerned with, among other things, self-preservation. This system is involved in the "fight-or-flight" response described in Chapters 2 and 6, when the neurotransmitter norepinephrine, which at normal levels helps us maintain our blood pressure and maintain alertness, is released in excessive quantities so we can defend ourselves or outrun a predator.

What makes human beings what we are, however, is the higher brain functions of reason, memory, morals, and so forth, which reside in the cerebral cortex.

Insomnia, as we are coming to know it, seems to involve one or all three nervous system components. Do you ever wake up in the middle of the night desperate for something to eat? That's the enteric nervous system in action.

Did you ever get so surprised by something that you vomited? Some people do. You could think of it as a combination of the autonomic nervous system and the enteric. If you experienced the insomnia of severe jet lag you probably felt the discomfort of the miscommunication between your gut and higher brain centers. The gastrointestinal system is one of the first to suffer in cases of severe jet lag.

Were you ever so worried about something that your stomach hurt? Your higher thought processes are hitting you in the gut.

Do you eat compulsively when you have to stay up all night? There is a connection between lack of sleep, weight gain, and the newly described hypocretin pathways, which will be discussed shortly.

Of course, not everything is a "gut" issue. Worries can keep you from falling asleep. The smallest sound can wake you up at night and not let you get back to sleep. There are infinite varieties of physical and mental combinations that can affect your sleeping adversely. The culmination of all this is something that is probably uniquely human, and that is, when the fear of sleeplessness itself keeps you awake at night. As far as we know, only humans can be afraid of an idea.

Responding to Stressors

Sometime in your family's very distant past, a jolt of norepinephrine may have saved one of your ancestors from a saber-toothed tiger. Let's face it, norepinephrine was one of those things that made the fittest fit enough to survive. That mechanism is still hardwired into our bodies. However, for most of the 24-hour day, it does routine duty helping regulate your day-night rhythms.

At night, secretion of norepinephrine throttles back to allow sleep to happen. However, modern life being stressful, there are many times during the day or night when something happens that provokes a jolt of norepinephrine. We call these things, understandably, "stressors." They can be real or imagined. They activate arousal mechanisms linked in the brain and body to the related fight-or-flight response. Needless to say, you don't want this to happen at bedtime. A stressor can be environmental, such as light, temperature, or noise; physical, such as pain; behavioral, such as exercise or a cigarette; psychological, such as an emotion or thought; and so on. Whatever the nature of a specific stressor, the body registers it in a way that can keep you awake. Stressors play a role in all types of insomnia, acute or chronic, primary or secondary, as we will see later on.

The Seeds of Cure

Dismal as insomnia can be, however, the seeds of cure may lie in our ability to master problems of both body and mind. Just as bullfighters are able to conquer their fears and children usually respond to a soothing bedtime routine, so we can teach ourselves to sleep again.

Hardwiring—Present Day

Some insomniacs are probably born, and some are made. Various studies show that insomniacs have higher body temperatures, greater frontalis muscle tension—tension in the muscles you massage in your temples—and higher electrical conductivity in their skin than noninsomniacs, which may help us understand why insomniacs are so sensitive to changes in room temperature.

A recent study used PET scan imaging to compare brain glucose consumption in insomniacs to that of normal sleepers. The insomniac group clearly had more brain sugar consumption and activity throughout most of the brain during wake and sleep. Evidence also points to this continued state of chronic insomnia as associated with altered immunity and disease.

However, whether we are hardwired for insomnia or not, we are also prone to certain kinds of behavior that can lead to insomnia. This is because the sleep-wake cycle is also hardwired into our bodies, as it is in the bodies of most large creatures. The brain is, of course, command central: home to 100 billion nerve cells, an estimated quadrillion connections and trillions of support cells that send signals over an incredibly complex superhighway to every muscle and organ system in the body. The hallmark of this system is its regularity. Hormones and neurotransmitters are secreted in a way that meets the demands of the 24-hour day on a caveman's schedule, which was programmed by sunlight. The autonomic nervous system, for example, secretes enough norepinephrine to maintain our blood pressure and heartbeat at levels necessary to sustain normal daytime activity and then reduces activity during sleep.

Of course, the nervous system also has plenty of emergency capacity, and in modern society we routinely abuse that capacity, both voluntarily and involuntarily.

Some of us do it for a living. Professional wrestlers work themselves into a frenzy, accompanied by pounding hearts and veins sticking out in their necks and foreheads, by inducing a surge in the same norepinephrine that keeps us on our feet and alert. The effect on the audience may be theatrical, but the effects on the wrestlers' bodies are very real.

The rest of us don't routinely work ourselves up into a froth the way the Pay-per-View gladiators do. Instead we worry, lose our tempers in traffic, obsess about our jobs, and fight to get by on six hours of sleep when we really need eight. As anyone who has ever felt depressed after yelling at his or her spouse or children can attest, abuse of this system has its price. If we do it regularly, we are using up a physical resource that cannot be quickly or easily replaced. We are depleting key neurochemicals and perhaps altering the neuropathways we rely on to function on an inborn rhythmic schedule.

In the short run, our ability to sleep suffers. In the long run, there is the potential for damage to many other parts of the body. Our nervous system has not changed much over the last 10,000 years. It works great when left alone, but we have to read the manual to maintain it and fix it.

REPLACEMENT PARTS

We can replace most body parts using incredible technology, but so far there is no transplant for the central nervous system. When things go wrong, one of our most primitive needs is one of the first casualties: the need to sleep properly. When we disregard this critical need, the body and mind pay us back with discomfort, malfunction, and disease.

However, there is a new focus in sleep medicine to help both mind and body return to a natural rhythm of active by day and quiet by night.

We do this by using retraining and behavioral techniques, accompanied, when necessary, by medication. The mind responds well to retraining, and the body can be treated or repaired. A new and exciting group of medications designed to mimic our own nervous system transmitters are helping us repave pathways in the nervous system.

We are approaching, in effect, a neurochemical transplant designed to help our bodies and mind get back to the original design of circadian harmony. These are not the sleeping pills of old, with their reputation for addiction. Medications are getting so sophisticated that eventually, when used properly, they may be as precise as surgery. They will mimic or bridge our natural neurochemical pathways so that our bodies will be able to return to the schedule they are supposed to be on. A program of medication, accompanied by behavioral and cognitive therapy, which, as I will describe later, deals with *what we do* and *what we think,* can be compared to a program of surgery and rehabilitation with physical, speech, and occupational therapy. We are at the threshold of another frontier.

Another factor in the explanation of insomnia may involve a change in brain chemistry as a cause of some cases of insomnia. A study by Jerome M. Siegel, M.D., professor of psychiatry and a member of the Brain Research Institute at the UCLA Medical Center and chief of neurobiology research at the Sepulveda Veterans Affairs Medical Center, points to histamine and serotonin as well as norepinephrine.

The one with the most easily recognizable role is histamine. Those of you with allergies know all about this substance. It is present in mast cells, which are part of your immune system, and is released when you are exposed to allergens. Histamine makes you sneezy, itchy, and so on. That's why you take an antihistamine to relieve symptoms. What you may not have known is that there is histamine in your brain as well, and it is necessary for staying awake.

This also explains why a so-called first generation antihistamine like Benadryl is a sedative, whereas later generations such as Claritin and Allegra do not make you sleepy. The older drugs pass through the brain blood barrier and counteract the histamine in the brain, which is an essential part of your brain function. It's supposed to be there to help you stay awake.

"Catch a Wave"—Revisited

In Chapter 3, we discussed how normal sleep is like catching a wave and effortlessly riding it. The well-prepared surfer paddles out into the ocean and waits for the right wave.

For those with insomnia, that wave never arrives. They sit out there in the surf, the water rises and falls, but somehow that big one—the one they can ride straight through till morning—never comes along.

The problem may be as simple as a behavioral or lifestyle choice that you are loathe to give up, such as the ritual of an after-dinner cup of coffee or the habit of watching *The Tonight Show* on television, on the one hand, or as complex as divorce or a crisis of faith on the other. You may have an underlying physical or psychological tendency that combines with an ordinary event to throw you off your routine, and you can't regain your equilibrium.

Who Gets Insomnia?

The task of measuring how many of us have insomnia is compli-cated by the fact that many of us choose to live with our problems. If a tree falls in the forest and no one reports hearing it, does it make any noise?

How many of us choose to put up with our sleeplessness because we're afraid to admit that we have lost control over our lives or don't want to confront the underlying problems contributing to our sleep-lessness? How many of us self-medicate with warm baths, warm milk, alcohol, or over-the-counter sleep aids? How many of us won't "waste" a doctor's appointment on a "trivial" matter?

This is not just a tendency among busy Americans. A survey of five European countries (Britain, Sweden, Germany, Ireland, and Bel-gium) commissioned by life sciences group Rhone-Poulenc Rorer, showed that two out of three people in Britain suffer from insomnia, mostly linked to stress and personal worries. In Sweden the rate was even higher—75 percent. Germany had the lowest rate—"only" 45 percent of the population was affected. Women are more likely to suf-fer from sleepless nights than men.

As you might expect, the main reasons these people lie awake at night include health concerns and relationship difficulties. The survey found that severe insomniacs had often experienced marital break-downs or were single parents. The study also showed that in Britain and Sweden, those with difficulty going to sleep and waking frequently during the night were more likely to be in the 25–34 age bracket than any other.

A study by German researchers found that roughly 20–30 percent of adults worldwide suffer from insomnia, but estimated that fewer than 50 percent of them will be diagnosed with it, largely for the sim-ple reason that most never discuss it with a doctor.

The best estimates are that 10–12 percent of Americans are suffer-ing from insomnia at any one time, but that anywhere from 30–50 per-cent have bouts of insomnia in the course of a year. Again, we can't be sure because most cases never make it as far as a doctor's office.

Physical, Mental, and Emotional Impairment

Insomniacs are people who have problems getting to sleep or stay-ing asleep and as a result have physical, mental, or emotional impair-ment over an extended period of time. Insomnia is found in men and women of all age groups, although it seems to be more common in women (especially after menopause) and in the elderly. Contrary to conventional wisdom, it's the *ability* to sleep, rather than the *need* for sleep, that appears to decrease with advancing age.

Among nonelderly adult women, they are more likely to be home-makers than those who work in jobs, older rather than younger, and blue-collar rather than professional.

Insomnia Definitions
THE ROAD TO INSOMNIA

We all know what it's like to have an occasional sleepless night, or even several in a row. For most people, these are relatively unremark-able episodes. For insomniacs, however, these same events are the start of a long, dark journey.

Insomnia is a symptom defined as inability to fall asleep within 30 minutes, inability to stay asleep or waking up at the wrong time. In addition the insomnia events impact on your quality of life.

Some of these events are based on your senses and your thought processes or cognitive factors. "What happens if I don't sleep?" "How will lack of sleep affect my life?" These are examples of thoughts that can overwhelm an insomniac and prevent sleep from coming.

Others, such as anxiety, are emotive, which, as the term implies, stem from your underlying feelings such as a sense of inadequacy, sad-ness, anger, or resentment.

Still others are physiological, such as acid reflux.

Some happen at the beginning of your bedtime and interfere with your getting to sleep. This is referred to as sleep onset insomnia.

When you are awakened during one of the later phases of sleep by an event such as a noise, a nightmare, or tossing and turning by a rest-less bedmate and you find it difficult to get back to sleep, it is called sleep maintenance insomnia. There may also be a sleep state misper-ception disorder where you feel that sleep is restless or not deep enough but the subsequent sleep study shows that your sleep is just fine.

A **stressor,** a term mentioned earlier, can be any disturbing factor that wedges itself between the body-and-mind harmony. The stressor may be medical, environmental, or mental in origin. Since the nervous system works in both directions, receiving and sending signals, there are many different possible combinations of disruptive signaling sce-narios that can result in insomnia.

At New York Hospital, we are fortunate to have Arthur J. Spielman, Ph.D., as the director of our research division. A leader in the field of insomnia, he is responsible for contributing much to our knowledge of insomnia. His model of insomnia is taught to students at all levels, including doctoral-level students in training at our center. This model is summarized as follows:

1. *Predisposing factors*—traits, genetic or acquired, that make us less able to get to sleep or liable to be easily awakened. During the day, before they show up as part of insomnia, they may appear as anxious, obsessive, or compulsive behavior.

2. *Precipitating circumstances*—things that happen in our lives that make it hard for us to sleep. These can be both good things and bad things. The birth of a child would be a good thing that might set off a bout of insomnia. A bad thing—let's count them: death, accident, divorce, loss of a job. A change from day shift to night shift at work is also a precipitating factor that will adversely affect our sleep.

3. *Perpetuating factors*—the things that happen over a period of time that prolong the initial sleeplessness. For example, that initial joy at becoming a parent might be followed by a bout of colic, or a few months later by teething.

Any of these factors can bleed into one another.

TAKING THE MASK OFF THE MANY TIRED FACES OF INSOMNIA

People with insomnia also are mostly unaware that chronic insomnia is an established risk factor for psychiatric illness. Their risk of depression is four times greater than in those not suffering from sleeping difficulties. Part of the problem is doctors' training. In many medical schools, only 1.5 hours of teaching are devoted to the problem of insomnia.

Professor Jorge Alberto Costa E. Silva, of the New York University School of Medicine in New York City, has observed that physicians often overlook insomnia as a precursor of serious illness. He said, "Poor sleepers are more than twice as likely as good sleepers to have ischemic heart disease in the six years after first experiencing sleeping difficulties, and they are also about three times as likely as good sleepers to develop frequent headaches." People with insomnia are ambivalent about their own condition, and most do not discuss insomnia with their medical doctors. Each specialist focuses on disease in his or her own specific area of expertise and the effects of insomnia—a condition that affects the entire body—on that particular organ are often overlooked.

Most people experience insomnia at one time or another and eventually return to normal sleep patterns. It's not that they don't feel tired during the day, or yawn, or feel muscular discomfort. But they are able to return rapidly to circadian balance.

However, for those prone to or predisposed to chronic insomnia, the sleeplessness soon takes on a life of its own. They enter what psychologist Charles Morin calls "a vicious cycle of insomnia, emotional and cognitive arousal, and further sleep disturbances."

They come to associate their bedtime and bedroom with worry about being able to go to sleep. What should be a comforting process becomes about as welcome as the prospect of having a tooth pulled.

They develop a symptom we normally associate with another bedroom activity: performance anxiety. The more they try to sleep, the more difficult it gets. They try drinking warm milk and taking hot baths or drinking or reading or doing push-ups. The problem begins to snowball.

The fear of sleeplessness soon begins to throw them off their schedules. Don't forget, sleep comes in waves, and pretty soon, they begin to grab whatever wave comes along. They fall asleep watching TV or reading at 9:30 P.M., and are wide awake at 1:00 A.M. They fall asleep on the couch and not in bed. Then they go back to bed where their bed partner is sound asleep and disturb his or her sleep.

LIFE-CHANGING EVENTS

The inability to sleep is frequently combined with a life-changing event that is itself a shock to the system.

Public speaking coaches are fond of telling their pupils that getting up in front of an audience to give a speech is one of life's most stressful experiences, in company with dealing with the death of a loved one. This was borne out in a 1982 study in which subjects were told prior to taking a nap that they would have to give a speech after they woke up. These were good sleepers. Yet they took much longer to fall asleep than a control group who weren't so threatened.

I raise this point to show that anyone can have an insomnia attack if they are exposed to certain sources of stress. Whether this turns into chronic insomnia, however, is contingent on a much more extensive set of underlying factors, both psychological and physiological.

Other major stressors include job loss, moving to a new house, marriage, divorce—the list of life-changing events is very long.

Types of Insomnia

It is not possible to describe all types of insomnia with a single model, although there are several ways to think about insomnia. One way is *duration*.

A FEW DAYS TO SEVERAL WEEKS—ACUTE INSOMNIA—BAD THINGS COME TO AN END

Strange as this may sound, if you have transient or acute insomnia, you are one of the lucky ones. That said, if symptoms last for more than a few days, you should get some help.

The following are major contributors to acute insomnia:

• Stress
• Noise
• Extreme temperatures
• Change in the immediate environment
• Sleep/wake schedule problems such as those due to jet lag
• Side effects of medication

Treatment for transient insomnia, if needed, includes reassurance, supportive stress therapy, and occasionally a short course of a mild hypnotic. More treatment options are outlined below.

ONE TO SIX MONTHS—INTERMITTENT, OR OCCURRING MORE THAN THREE TIMES A WEEK

This is similar to acute insomnia in terms of the potential causes; however, by definition symptoms persist for a longer time. Treatment options are similar to those for acute insomnia with more emphasis on cognitive and behavioral therapy as time goes on. There is also a recent study demonstrating the safety of treating this type of insomnia with the newer hypnotics.

Chronic insomnia may be caused by many other chronic medical conditions or may be a primary insomnia, which, as described earlier, means that there is no easily identified disease or stressor. When sleep is disturbed for long enough, whether stressors are identifiable or not, your sleep routine is thrown off and the expectation that you will have difficulty sleeping becomes self-fulfilling. In an attempt to allay your anxiety or to cope with life in spite of it, you may develop some of these habits that violate the tenets of good sleep hygiene and may also contribute directly to chronic insomnia:

- Consuming too much coffee, cola drinks, or other sources of caffeine during the day, as well as close to bedtime
- Drinking alcohol before bedtime
- Smoking cigarettes before bedtime
- Afternoon naps or dozing after dinner
- Irregular sleep-wake schedules

Secondary Causes of Insomnia—Identifying Stressors

MEDICAL STRESSORS

Virtually any medical problem can cause insomnia, but the more prominent ones include heart or lung disease, allergies, arthritis, cancer, fibromyalgia, gastroesophageal reflux disease (GERD), hypertension, rheumatologic conditions, Alzheimer's disease, Parkinson's disease, hyperthyroidism, and attention deficit hyperactivity disorder.

MEDICATIONS AS STRESSORS

The medications we use can also disturb our sleep and aggravate our tendencies toward insomnia. Check the warnings and potential side effects of most over-the-counter cold remedies and you will see insomnia listed. Among the many other medications that can cause insomnia are antidepressants (e.g., fluoxetine, bupropion), theophylline, beta-blockers, asthma medications, nicotine, and, of course, caffeine.

Chronic insomnia is frequently associated with psychologic or psychiatric disorders. The disorders that most often cause insomnia, in order of frequency, are:

- Anxiety
- Depression (more than 90 percent of depressed patients experience insomnia)
- Bipolar disorder

Insomnia may *cause* emotional problems, and it is often unclear which came first.

SUBSTANCE-ABUSE STRESSORS

Chronic insomnia is frequently a result of substance abuse. Alcohol, cocaine, sedatives, and hypnotics may cause disrupted sleep. One or two alcoholic drinks a day, for most people, pose little danger of serious side effects and may actually offer some protection against heart disease. Excess alcohol, however, or alcohol used to promote sleep, suppresses REM sleep and tends to fragment sleep and cause wakefulness a few hours later. Alcohol and any sedating medication also increase the risk for other sleep disorders, including sleep apnea and restless legs. Alcoholics often suffer insomnia and REM sleep behavior disorders.

SHIFT WORK STRESSORS

Shift workers often have insomnia, and shift-work sleep disorder is discussed in detail in Chapter 15.

ADDITIONAL STRESSORS FOR SECONDARY INSOMNIA

Among the elderly and patients with psychiatric disorders, certain stress hormones are *persistently elevated.* Cortisol in particular is elevated at night in the elderly and may affect REM sleep. Normal aging is associated with a blunting of regular, cyclical surges of growth hormone, which is normally secreted in the late night and is associated not only with growth but with deep, slow-wave sleep.

Insomnia may have a genetic component, since approximately 35 percent of people with insomnia have a family history of the condition, with the mother being the most commonly affected family member.

SLEEP DISORDERS AS A CAUSE OF INSOMNIA

Any sleep disorder can cause secondary insomnia. The disturbances of RLS (Chapter 9), obstructive sleep apnea (Chapters 6 and 7), or shift-work sleep disorders (Chapter 15) are enough to prod us into wakefulness.

Treatment of Secondary Insomnia

A college student came to see me at the sleep center for a complaint of insomnia that had lasted for a year. His mother had insomnia, but although he had had only occasional problems with sleep, the pattern of not falling asleep did not set in until his first year of college when he would regularly go to bed at 1 to 3 A.M. After the initial visit and evaluation at the sleep center, we identified moderate obesity, severe allergic rhinitis, enlarged adenoids and tonsils, hyperthyroidism, caffeine abuse (up to six cups of coffee per day to help him in his studies), poor sleep habits developing over the year, and anxiety related to his academic performance.

Over the next four months all of the medical, sleep, and psychiatric issues causing the secondary insomnia were addressed, along with a caffeine-free weight-loss diet and a new attitude about sleep. One year later he is back on the dean's list and sleeping well.

Primary Insomnia—No Identifiable Stressors

If all of the causes of secondary insomnia are ruled out after a complete review at the sleep center, then you are considered to have a primary insomnia. Whether we find a cause of the disorder or not, the consequences are very real. Insomnia and the associated daytime sleepiness results in impaired social, occupational, physical, and intellectual functioning. Common features of primary insomnia include increased mortality in short sleepers; increased risk of depression, anxiety, substance abuse, and nicotine dependence; and worrying about insomnia to the point where it diminishes your enjoyment of life in general. Primary insomnia accounts for about 15 percent of all insomnia cases referred to sleep centers; it is more common in women than men, and can occur at any age. Of all patients with chronic insomnia 25 percent have primary insomnia.

The term *primary insomnia* is not accepted by all doctors and some prefer to consider it as one of the following:

Psychophysiologic insomnia. This describes the vicious cycle of stress, "trying too hard to sleep," and bad habits that make the problem worse.

Idiopathic insomnia. Idiopathic (meaning no known cause) insomnia is a lifelong sleeplessness, which may be attributed to a neurological abnormality in the sleep/wake center of the brain, for which there is no known remedy.

Sleep state misperception. A disorder in which the patient reports insomnia but the evaluations including sleep studies are normal.

General Treatment Approach to All Types of Insomnia

In treating insomnia, it is helpful to consider it in terms of the final mind-body complaint. If you have insomnia, there is usually disharmony among the three components of sound sleep: mind, body, and the nervous system. The sleep complaint will involve one or any combination of these three components, often with an indistinct connection to the insomnia, as in the case of a medication effect or excessive caffeine. The initial evaluation is the first step in identifying correctable mind, body, or nervous system stressors.

FIRST VISIT TO THE SLEEP CENTER

Considering the complex nature of insomnia and the many potential causes, the initial evaluation is extremely important in pointing the way to proper diagnosis and treatment. The evaluation often begins before you see the doctor. Most sleep centers do a screening and ask the patient to complete questionnaires and sleep diaries prior to the first visit. This information can be completed in the waiting room or mailed in ahead of the visit. Other components of the evaluation include a complete medical, psychiatric, and sleep history.

The Physical Exam

A physical examination must be done in order to properly evaluate a complaint of insomnia. It may reveal, for example, a thyroid mass or nodule or neurological disease which may explain the complaint quite neatly. Carefully directed blood work or radiological tests may also add to the diagnosis of a secondary sleep disorder or help confirm a primary insomnia.

When this evaluation is complete and all necessary testing is done, a diagnosis and treatment plan follow. All secondary stressors and conditions are addressed. If the insomnia persists, treatments continue as outlined below.

STOP SELF-MEDICATION—IT'S DANGEROUS AND INEFFECTIVE

The first resort of people with insomnia is often to attempt to fix the problem themselves. One study showed that Americans spent as much on non-prescription drugs and alcohol for insomnia as they did on health care services and medications: nearly $14 billion. This trend of self-medication is incredibly dangerous. While sleeping pills must be prescribed by a physician, which implies that the physician monitors the patient's dosage and administration, long-term usage must be managed carefully. Self-medicating with alcohol is not only dangerous and unhealthy, but counterproductive to attaining restful sleep.

A recent study found that a significant number of patients initially complaining of insomnia actually had an undiagnosed sleep apnea and other sleep disorders. Indeed, at our sleep center, about one in five patients who complain of insomnia are found to warrant a sleep study based on our initial evaluation. Out of this group, the majority are found to have significant sleep disorders other than insomnia that require a specific treatment.

No chapter in a book could possibly do justice to the full range of factors that contribute to insomnia. Beyond those we have just discussed, precipitating and perpetuating factors can include physical disease such as arthritis and chronic fatigue syndrome, kidney failure and heart failure, and menopause. They can include psychological and psychiatric conditions, such as depression and anxiety, psychosis and schizophrenia. They can be environmental or induced by responses to external factors. Each requires a careful initial first step: diagnosis. Treating an underlying disease is the most important first step in treating insomnia. Resorting to medication in order to deal with the symptoms of insomnia can mask another problem and exacerbate your medical condition over the long run.

However, there's one thread that does run through the treatment of all types of insomnia, and that is the thread of your daily routine, your sleep hygiene, which I discussed in Chapter 3, and which I'll address below.

Acute and intermittent insomnia treatments. Acute insomnia often resolves itself when a stressful situation is resolved. Treatments were discussed on page 175.

Chronic insomnia treatments. A wide range of behavioral, non-pharmacologic and pharmacologic treatments are available for all types of chronic insomnia.

As a seasoned insomniac, I knew sometimes the way to beat sleeplessness was to outwit it: to pretend you didn't care about sleeping. Then sometimes sleep became piqued, like a rejected lover, and crept up to try to seduce you.

—Erica Jong, *Fear of Flying*

Not all of us are as resourceful as Ms. Jong. We cannot "outwit" our insomnia without focusing on all the measures for healthy living: exercise, diet, and sleep. Sleep hygiene measures as simple as eliminating caffeine after noon can actually cure insomnia. I had a 19-year-old patient who didn't realize that the two liters of cola soda he drank while he studied could be a cause of his eight-month insomnia jag. You may think this is "obvious," but I see such "obvious" mistakes very often in my practice.

Nicotine and medication side effects are other common contributors. Environmental factors such as light, noise, temperature, and mattress comfort may be important. A program of sleep hygiene education should be a necessary part of all interventions, behavioral or pharmacological.

When there is no clear cause for the insomnia and the problem has become chronic, other treatments are needed. Medication is not the first line of therapy for the chronic insomnias, although when the symptoms are severe in terms of either the effects on the body or psyche, a short course of medication may be helpful.

Behavioral therapy helps you develop tools to assist you in reaching specific goals and gain more control over your life. Examples of sleep goals include: Things you *do,* such as using the bedroom only for sleep; how you *feel,* such as changing your body's response to stress; what you *think,* such as getting over the idea that you don't need that much sleep if you are elderly; and *managing* skills, such as changing the ways you cope with medical illness.

Behavioral therapy for sleep starts with good sleep hygiene and daytime behavior that prepares you for a good night's sleep. Preparing your mind and body by staying mentally and physically healthy is a good first step for any endeavor, sleep included. The following is list of behavioral therapy techniques that might help alleviate insomnia.

1. *Stimulus control.* The objective is to train the person with insomnia to reassociate the bed and bedroom with rapid sleep onset. Examples include not watching TV in bed, not balancing the checkbook in bed, and not having a long emotional conversation on the phone while lying in bed. This method helps when there is a learned or conditioned response associating the bed and bedroom with poor sleep.

2. *Progressive muscle relaxation.* These techniques involve tensing and relaxing different muscle groups throughout the body. This therapy was developed to help insomnia patients who often display high levels of arousal both at night and during the day.

3. *Paradoxical intention.* This method involves persuading a patient to engage in his or her most feared behavior, i.e., staying awake. The goal is to eliminate performance anxiety, as it may inhibit sleep onset. Due to variability of response, it is not clear which insomnia types might respond to this approach.

4. *Biofeedback.* Biofeedback operates on the idea that we can influence certain automatic body functions by using our minds. Once thought to be "science fiction," biofeedback has proven its effectiveness in reducing stress-related physiological symptoms. Sensors that record muscle contractions and skin temperature, for example, can help a patient learn to control involuntary processes such as heart rate and blood pressure,

which increase under stress. By "feeding back" physiological measures, which are registered on EEG-type monitors, you can learn to recognize and control facets of stress. Biofeedback techniques can be effective in treating migraine headaches, asthma, and other disorders.

5. *Sleep restriction.* This technique was developed by Dr. Spielman and is very helpful for some patients. Time in bed is carefully controlled and limited in order to help consolidate sleep and improve sleep efficiency.

6. *Multicomponent cognitive and behavioral therapy.* This type of therapy may include combinations of both psychological and behavioral methods, aimed at changing the patient's beliefs and attitudes about insomnia in addition to methods such as stimulus control, sleep restriction, or progressive muscle relaxation as previously described.

7. *Sleep hygiene education.* As mentioned, this form of behavioral intervention seeks to make patients more aware of beneficial health practices that affect sleep, such as proper diet, adequate exercise, and avoidance of substance abuse; and of environmental factors such as light, noise, and temperature control, and choice of mattress. Sleep hygiene education is often included with other behavioral interventions such as multicomponent cognitive behavioral therapy described above.

8. *Imagery training.* This treatment involves visualizing or focusing on pleasant or neutral images. Examples include guiding and teaching a person to imagine a pleasant walk on a beach or other calming real-life experiences. This may be considered a subcategory of relaxation therapy. Counting sheep was probably the original version of this technique, although some may consider it too exciting.

9. *Cognitive therapy.* Cognitive therapy helps correct faulty beliefs and attitudes about sleep. The therapist and patient will work out a strategy that is suited to the individual from a growing number of specific techniques. Specific examples may include an effort to stop taking sleeplessness so seriously and to defuse a patient's obsessions with the night that have crowded out day-

time thinking. By emphasizing one's daytime preoccupations, we can help diminish the cycle of apprehension about sleeplessness and the accompanying emotional stress, dysfunctional cognitions, and disturbed sleep itself.

MEDICATION FOR INSOMNIA

I said above that our sleep center prefers to treat insomnia without medication. It is also true that I prescribe medication to patients every week. This is not a contradiction in practice but rather a mind-body rescue. Since insomnia can be so debilitating, we need to help get the person back to a healthy state of mind and body as quickly as possible.

The list of medications for insomnia is long and, as with any medication, there are always concerns about side effects. Several medications have stood the test of time in my practice, namely Ambien and some of the benzodiazepines. I use them for very specific types of insomnia, however, and use them with great caution in patients with serious medical conditions including those with secondary insomnia from severe heart and/or lung disease. We need more clinical research on the safety of these and the newer insomnia medications on patients with medical and sleep disorders and secondary insomnia.

THE STRAIGHT DOPE ON SLEEPING PILLS

Sleeping pills have gotten a bad rap over many years. To many people, the term still conjures up visions of long-term dependency and Marilyn Monroe. The good news is that we have come a long way since the days of phenobarbitol and tranquilizers like Miltown; we are living better through chemistry.

Not only are today's drugs generally better, due to our superior knowledge of how the brain works, but we also have very precise knowledge of their efficacy and thus the limits of their effectiveness.

That is not to say that they can't be abused. The efficacy of any drug depends largely on compliance, with the rules spelled out by the manufacturer and the physician.

Pharmaceutical Insomnia Treatments

Class of drug	Nonprescription drugs	Benzodiazepine Hypnotics	Nonbenzodiazepine Hypnotics	Antidepressants
Brand names	Benadryl, BayerPM, ExcedrinPM, Nytol, Sominex, Unisom	Restoril, Dalmane, ProSom, Halcion	Ambien, Sonata	Elavil, Endep, Enovil
Active ingredients, and how they work	Antihistamines, which penetrate brain blood barrier and suppress mediator histamine, crucial for wakefulness	Benzodiazepines (BZDs), which enhance GABA neurotransmission, resulting in sedation, muscle relaxation, anxiolysis, and anticonvulsant effects	Zolpidem and zaleplon, which work on same parts of brain as BZDs, but have faster absorption, metabolism, and elimination	Tricyclic antidepressant groups Serotonin reuptake inhibitors
Duration of use	10–14 days, but with limited effectiveness after two or three	7–10 days	7–10 days	**Last choice and usually to help depression symptoms**
Advantages and disadvantages	Diminished quality of sleep because of limited REM sleep	Alter REM and non-REM sleep, addictive if used for too long, and deadly in combination with alcohol	Shorter-lasting side effects than BZDs; may be preferable for insomnia patients who need to be alert due to societal or occupational demands, who may have to wake up in a few hours, or who suffer from sleep-onset insomnia	Nonaddictive although possible to overdose; doubtful effectiveness; recommended only in cases where depression must be treated
Side Effects	Antihistamines are also used for allergy relief; thus you may also experience side effects associated with the sinuses, inner ear, and mouth: dry mouth, next-day grogginess, dizziness, headache, and coordination problems	Next-day hangovers, grogginess, slurring of speech, and diminished coordination; Halcion linked to depression, amnesia, anxiety, and hallucinations	Same as BZDs, but much less severe	Dry mouth, heart arrhythmias

Class of drug	Nonprescription drugs	Benzodiazepine Hypnotics	Nonbenzodiazepine Hypnotics	Antidepressants
What the doctors say	Avoid use in treating sleep disorders	These drugs were created in 1960 and like most first-generation drugs, they reflect how little scientists and doctors knew about them. They are not first-line therapy but are still used with caution in some cases.	First-line therapy when medication is needed; nonpharmacologic methods preferred	Not first-line therapy for most sleep disorders

"Natural" Remedies		
Type of Drug	Melatonin	Herbal Remedies
What is it?	Hormone produced in the brain which helps regulate sleep-wake cycle	Forms of plants such as valerian, chamomile, lemon balm, lavender, hops, passionflower, and kava, which contain compounds thought to promote sleep
Forms of administration	Natural and artificial supplements available in health food stores and drugstores without prescriptions	Teas, supplements, extracts
Projected benefits	Treating sleep disturbances caused by jet lag, shift work, and other disruption of the biological clock	Rain forest remedies on the horizon?
Does it work?	Short-term use for jet lag is the most effective use; long-term benefits unproven	Unproven by scientific methods. "Proof" often anecdotal and folkloric
Warnings	Quality control: Real dosages often differ from those on labels; organic melatonin is taken from cattle brains, and thus may spread mad cow disease, although the odds are long. Ask a pharmacist to recommend a reputable brand.	Many poisons are "natural." Socrates, the philosopher was executed by being forced to drink hemlock. Some of these supplements may be harmless. Kava has been linked by the FDA to extreme liver damage.
What the doctor says	Needs more research. Might be part of a combination pill in the future.	Caution. Any chemical or substance put into the body the wrong way can be harmful.

Action of Medications Used in the Treatment of Insomnia

Agent	Dosage	Peak Action	Half-life
Estazolam (ProSom)	1–2 mg	2 hours (0.5–6 hours)	10–24 hours
Flurazepam (Dalmane)	15–30 mg	0.5–1 hour	2–3 hours (47–100 hours for metabolite)
Oxazepam (Serax)	10–15 mg	3 hours	5–10 hours
Quazepam (Doral)	7.5–15 mg	2 hours	41 hours (47–100 hours for metabolite)
Temazepam (Restoril)	7.5–30 mg	1.2–1.6 hours	3.5–18.4 hours (9–15 hours for metabolite)
Triazolam (Halcion)	0.125–0.5 mg	1–2 hours	1.5–5.5 hours
Zolpidem (Ambien)	5–10 mg	1.6 hours	2.5 hours

Future Drugs* for Treatment of Insomnia

Drug	How It Works	Comments
Ambien CR (Zolpidem MR)	Non-benzodiazepine GABA-A modulator	Available now in shorter-acting form. See above.
Gaboxadol	GABA-A agonist	Works on GABA-A receptors
Indiplon IR, Indiplon MR	GABA-A modulator	Works on GABA-A receptors
Lunesta (Eszopiclone)	Non-benzodiazepine GABA-A modulator	Similar drug used in Europe for over 10 years
Ramelteon	Melatonin receptor agonist	Work on receptors in the brain's master clock in suprachiasmatic nuclei (SCN)
Sonata (Zaleplon) extended-release	GABA-A modulator	Available now in shorter-acting form. See above.
Valdoxan (Agomelatine)	5-HT2C antagonist, 5-HT2B antagonist, melatonin receptor agonist	For use in depression, anxiety and sleep disorders

*Drugs currently in different phases of clinical trials and /or review by the FDA for use in treating insomnia.

Treating Neuropathways with "Future Drugs"

GABA (gamma-aminobutyric acid) is an inhibitory neurotransmitter, which means that when it finds its way to its receptor sites, it blocks the tendency of that neuron or nerve cell to fire. GABA slows down the excitatory neurotransmitters, like norepinephrine, that lead to anxiety. If you have too little GABA, you may tend to suffer from anxiety disorders. It is also one of the neurotransmitters released in the biochemical cycle that is thought to initiate sleep onset. Drugs that enhance GABA will have a sedating effect.

Norepinephrine (formerly called noradrenaline), is associated with, among other things, the fight-or-flight response discussed in the beginning of this chapter. It brings our nervous system into red alert in response to stressors and is prevalent in the sympathetic nervous system.

The new class of hypnotic medications work by enhancing GABA-like action, slowing down the effects of noreadrenaline, or by blocking some of the norepinephrine action. There are currently six or seven other drugs in the early phases of development that work on pathways involved in control of sleep such as the histamine and serotonin pathways.

The newer medications have very specific modes of action and are getting closer and closer to mimicking the action of our natural sleep-regulating neurotransmitters. GABA-A receptor agonists (non-benzodiazepines) are currently the cornerstone for the treatment of insomnia. However, the development of several other new medications, some of which are listed above, over the next three years will help expand our choices to match the equally diverse and often complex profiles and problems of insomnia patients.

Melatonin, for example, is known to participate in the sleep-wake cycle, although to date problems with quality and dose control have limited its usefulness. There is a new class of drugs that act on the melatonin receptors in the SCN (which was described earlier as being the biologic clock region of the brain), and we hope they will be more predictable than the over-the-counter preparations.

Benzodiazepines have been the gold standard for the treatment of insomnia and continue to be very useful in treating some cases of insomnia. However, because of their potential for pharmacologic dependence and withdrawal reactions upon discontinuation, they are neither recommended nor FDA-approved for treatment of chronic insomnia.

Zopiclone has been used in Europe for some time and appears to be well tolerated. Eszopiclone is a very similar preparation that has been studied for long-term use and is available for treating chronic insomnia in the United States.

All of the newer agents will expand the list of medications available that, when necessary, can be added to cognitive behavioral therapy as part of the total treatment for insomnia.

Tales of Two Retirements

There is one major contributing factor to insomnia that we can do nothing about—getting older. Insomnia is common among people over the age of 60. It's not that they need less sleep, but rather that they have more trouble getting it. Retirement is one of those life-changing events mentioned earlier in this chapter, and it's going to loom very large in the practice of sleep medicine as tens of millions of baby boomers reach retirement age. Retirement is an enormous adjustment both for those who don't have enough money saved for their later years and for those who do. Even the most avid golfer—and I deem myself among them—can only spend so much time on the course. The simple fact of the matter is that there *is* such a thing as too much of a good thing.

Retirement can be a real jolt to your ability to sleep through the night. But whether this jolt turns into a chronic problem depends on many other factors.

MY DAD

Like many retirees, my own father's sleep suffered when he stopped working. After 45 years as a butcher he found himself with long days with nothing to do. My mom still worked part-time and had her own hobbies and interests. His children and his grandchildren had their own lives to live.

What did the doctor order? This was clearly not a case where chemical intervention was warranted, even on a short-term basis. His health was good and there was nothing physically or mentally wrong with him. What he needed was something to help him pass the time, since his busy work schedule was no longer there to anchor him to his sleep-wake schedule. What he needed, in short, was a hobby.

In the end, the prescription was for a dose of Lhasa apso. I went to the pet store on Christmas Eve and bought Caesar. They have been constant companions for five years, and there was a dramatic improvement in my dad's daytime activity. As a consequence of his healthier and more active days, he enjoys healthier and more restful nights.

KATHERINE A.

In Chapter 2 I mentioned a former executive secretary. Katherine A. retired at about the same time as my father, and like him, she experienced a bout of insomnia. However, unlike my father's, hers lasted a long time and required much more complex treatment.

Katherine's life was about as different from my father's as you can get. She set out very early in life to pursue a career in ballet. She moved to New York in the late 1950s at the age of 16 to join one of the world-class ballet companies headquartered in the city.

Ballet training is rigorous. For Katherine, the demands of training and performance generally didn't leave much time for what we might consider a well-rounded existence.

Injured in her early 20s, Katherine had to find a way to make a living in the big city. The quickest route was to take a secretarial course. Smart and very disciplined, she got a job as secretary to an associate with a prominent law firm and rose through the ranks with him until he became an operating partner.

Being an executive secretary is a consuming occupation. When you combine that normally intense activity with the explosive growth of securities law in the late 20th century and the racehorse temperament of the former dancer, there wasn't much time left for anything but work until she retired. Take away those 10 hours a day or more of devotion to work and there's a tremendous void. Katherine felt a sense of emptiness that would take more than a pet to fill. She was depressed.

She got active in a church and in book groups, but there was no way that a patchwork of activities could substitute for the pattern of commitment that had been hers since her childhood, first as a dancer and then as executive secretary to a powerful and demanding boss.

Treating her insomnia initially required a combination of medication and both behavioral and cognitive therapy. Dr. Andrew Tucker, the associate director of our sleep center, decided on an initial trial of a **hypnotic** (sleeping pill), and an antidepressant aimed at reversing the sleep deficit and generally elevating her moods. Dosages of the medicines were slowly decreased over two to three months as the cognitive and behavioral therapy took effect. The therapy was a longer-term proposition. Recent studies have shown that a combination of cognitive and behavioral therapy is most successful in treating insomnia patients. The cognitive therapy initially aimed at getting her to recognize the deficits in the life she had lived, then to internalize her insights until she began to realize that she could derive fulfillment from her new life. The behavioral aspect of her therapy focused on improving her sleep hygiene, and getting her into the habit of preparing for a healthy night's sleep. Katherine has since returned to her previous energetic and productive self, using minimal medication.

Don't Let Insomnia Dominate Your Life

In his novel *One Hundred Years of Solitude,* Nobel Prize–winning author Gabriel Garcia Marquez writes about a "plague of insomnia." As the plague wears on, people lose their memory—they resort to leaving notes all over their homes to remind them how to function day-to-day. Even the most routine habits of life are forgotten. Their identities slip away. This literary invention seems the product of someone who has experienced prolonged inability to sleep. It is chronic insomnia taken to absurd lengths. For our purposes, however, it serves as a warning. Whatever the subtleties of your body chemistry or mental and physical response, your sleeplessness must be addressed. Predisposing, precipitating, and perpetuating factors reinforce one another. Left untreated, chronic sleeplessness comes to dominate your waking life, making it all you think about.

No single book or part of a book can help one cope with all manifestations of insomnia. There are many causes and the list keeps growing. What all of them have in common, however, is the advertent or inadvertent mismanagement of the biological clock. Not all people with insomnia will be capable of treating themselves. Not all professional treatment will be short-term, and it may require a mix of talk, behavioral, cognitive, and chemical therapies. By the time insomnia is diagnosed, the predisposing, precipitating, and perpetuating factors will be closely intertwined. As you've seen, some of these may be rooted in the most fundamental aspects of an individual's identity. For those, the question "Why can't I sleep?" probably can't definitively be answered without answering the question "Who am I, 24 hours a day?"

I am not a philosopher, nor am I a psychologist or a psychiatrist. The way I look at it, you have to start somewhere, and that is with the one thing that is out of kilter in every case of sleep disorder: the rhythm of a full 24-hour day and subsequently a good life.

Chronic insomnia is usually not "cured." What I tell my patients is that in all likelihood there will be *some* improvement. Many are satisfied by the end of a program combining medication, sleep hygiene, and behavioral and cognitive therapies; they will not only sleep better but have a better outlook on the entire 24-hour day. The take-home lesson is the recognition and acceptance that acute insomnia is a common and very temporary condition. We all have experienced it at one time or another, and since life is by definition occasionally stressful, to have an occasional sleepless night or a series of them is a fact of life.

I hope that after reading this chapter it is clear that when insomnia goes beyond that occasional night, it is time to get help. If several weeks pass and you still can't sleep, tell your doctor. Avoid chronic insomnia the way you would avoid a heart attack, a car accident, cancer, or the plague.

11

"AROUND SLEEP"—THE MYSTERIES OF PARASOMNIAS

Para is a Greek word that means "around" or "alongside." We use forms of it all the time—a *para*legal is someone who works with lawyers; *para*llel lines run alongside or around other lines at an equal distance; a slight variation on the root, *par*ody, is a creative work based on another work, and so on.

Parasomnia refers to a behavior or condition that takes place around or alongside sleep that has nothing to do with the central purpose of sleep and in fact detracts from it.

Life has traditionally been seen as divided into two states, waking and sleeping. From reading this book, you now know that it is actually three states—waking, non-REM sleep, and REM sleep.

Yet, there has always been a recognition, both from the "inside" and the "outside," that there was more to it than that. We know from the inside that the sleeping state can be rich with stories, characters, and ideas. People who could bring these thoughts to the rest of us were known variously as prophets, visionaries, and artists—that is, until the advent of psychoanalysis, at which point they were called therapists and patients. We also know from the outside that sleeping people are capable of some pretty bizarre behavior. For many centuries, men and women have watched and listened to their loved ones as they slept and wondered about their secret dreams.

With the advent of sleep medicine, the understanding of both the inner working script of the dream world and the witnessed outer performance of that script has increased dramatically. We know that dreaming is a function of REM sleep. As for that mysterious acting out, which we place under the umbrella term parasomnia, we now know that it is the result of confusion among the three states of existence—waking, the various stages of non-REM sleep, and REM sleep.

To understand parasomnias, it might help to review the descriptions of sleep stages from page 20 in Chapter 2. In stage 1, we drift into sleep and are easily reawakened; as we sink deeper into sleep, our eyes move very slowly and our muscle activity slows. In stage 2, our eye movements stop and brain waves slow down, with occasional bursts of rapid waves.

Remember, physical and mental processes begin to change during these two stages. People don't remember getting phone calls or other interruptions that take place. Nor do they remember turning off their alarms in the morning as they emerge from sleep.

In stage 3, extremely slow brain waves called delta waves appear in greater numbers, interspersed with smaller, faster waves. In stage 4, the brain switches to producing even more delta waves. This, along with stage 3, is referred to as deep sleep. It is very difficult to wake someone during stages 3 and 4.

During deep sleep, there is minimal eye movement or muscle activity. When awakened, people do not adjust immediately and often feel groggy and disoriented.

REM Sleep

In stage 5, our breathing speeds up and becomes irregular and shallow. Our eyes jerk rapidly in various directions—hence the name **rapid eye movement.** Our arm and leg muscles become temporarily paralyzed, our heart rate and blood pressure fluctuate, and there is an increased flow of blood to both male and female genitalia.

This takes place at intervals during the night.

Which State Am I In?

As with many other sleep disorders, we divide parasomnias into primary and secondary classifications. Primary parasomnias are categorized by the sleep states in which they occur. Behaviors reflect activation of the autonomic nervous system or disorders of movement or both. Sleepwalking in an otherwise healthy child is an example of a primary parasomnia.

Secondary parasomnias are defined as disorders of other organ systems that show up in sleep as a particular behavior or symptom. A particular disorder of the body, mind, or nervous system is directly contributing to the parasomnia. Examples include parasomnias associated with seizures, headaches, asthma, sleep-related abnormal swallowing syndrome, or respiratory-related confusional arousals. To the concerned parent, spouse, or family member, the nighttime behaviors associated with these secondary parasomnias may look just like the behavior seen in primary insomnia. Obviously the distinction between primary and secondary is one that influences the approach to treatment. If there is an identifiable underlying secondary cause, it must be treated. The behavior may or may not require additional treatments.

All parasomnias, whether primary or secondary, can be best understood as a malfunctioning of the switches that direct the timing, duration, and blending of the three states. In some parasomnias the sleep state may change rapidly and usually without warning, like a slow moving pinball bouncing between three major poles: awake . . . to REM . . . to non-REM. The patient's outward behavior and body action reflects all the bells and whistles of a 2-million-point bonus score; unfortunately, however, sometimes accompanied by more severe consequences for the patient or bed partner.

According to one classification scheme, all parasomnias are grouped under four categories: arousal disorders, sleep-wake transition disorders, REM sleep parasomnias, and other parasomnias.

Arousal Disorders

Arousal disorders are presumed to be related to a malfunction of the "wake to sleep switch." This can occur in the transition from wake to sleep or, most commonly, from deep sleep to wake. If you've ever tried to wake someone from deep sleep, you know basically what's involved: mental confusion and disorientation, resistance to being awakened, retrograde amnesia, or the inability to remember what happens, and so forth.

Arousal disorders themselves come in a number of varieties:

Confusional arousals. These are characterized by confusion during and after arousal from sleep, usually deep sleep, although without sleepwalking or sleep terrors. They generally are seen in young children. Subjects awaken only partially, start thinking slowly, and are disoriented about where they are and what time it is. Their perceptions are impaired. It can also be induced by anything that deepens sleep, such as sleep deprivation, and drugs that depress the central nervous system.

Sleep terrors. The patient awakens from slow-wave sleep with a piercing scream or cry, accompanied by tachycardia, or rapid heartbeat, sweating, shaking, and showing other physical and behavioral signs of intense fear. This usually takes place first around 90 minutes after sleep onset.

A test called a polysomnogram, or PSG, which records breathing and heart rate among other measures, reveals that people with sleep terrors often show a tendency for changes in heart rate throughout the night, and general arousal during other sleep stages.

Night terrors can be very disturbing to witness. It's difficult for parents to stand by and see their beloved child going through an intense physiologic autonomic response, consisting of pounding pulse, pouring sweat, red face, screaming, crying, and incoherent speech. An episode might last for five or ten minutes, which can seem like an eternity to a concerned parent. No wonder then that in the olden days this behavior was attributed to possession by a spirit.

But the olden days were not all that old. I had night terrors as a child. My grandfather, an immigrant ironworker, told my parents to throw water on me. When that didn't work, he told them to spell my name backward.

Like most sleep disorders, parasomnias have a strong tendency to run in families. While I never had a chance to ask my grandfather about it after I became interested in sleep medicine, I assume that someone in his family in the old country had night terrors and my forebears asked around for a "cure," hence his advice to my parents.

Fortunately for me, my worried parents took me to a good pediatrician who informed them that my terrors were harmless and that I would outgrow them. This set all their minds at ease, although I have had recurring but infrequent parasomnia episodes over the years. I shared a bedroom with my brothers and when we were teenagers, they got great fun out of watching me sit up in bed and ordering hamburgers, or driving a car and occasionally, in a panic, rooting around the foot of the bed for the brake because I thought I was going to crash. The last such reported episode happened during my first year of medical residency. My wife woke up and found me staring at one hand, mumbling about low oxygen levels and carbon-dioxide narcosis. The event reflected the combination of a difficult problem that day at the hospital diagnosing an elderly woman patient and the fact that like many residents, I was sleep deprived.

SLEEPWALKING, OR SOMNABULISM

Sleepwalking consists of a series of complex behaviors that start during slow-wave sleep. An estimated 18 percent of the population are prone to sleepwalking, and more of these sleepwalkers are young children rather than adolescents and adults. Boys are more likely to sleepwalk than girls. Sleepwalking is most common in children 11 to 12 years of age. Children who begin to sleepwalk at the age of nine often continue to do so into adulthood.

Episodes generally last from one to five minutes. The sleepwalker is usually very hard to awaken, seems confused when awakened, and has no memory of the episode. Here again, the disorder runs in families, and there may also be a personal and family history of other arousal disorders.

FIT TO BE TIED?

As I observed above, sleep disorders run in families. My sister was a sleepwalker. But never do to a child or adult for that matter what my father—out of genuine concern for her safety and on the advice of the family doctor—did to my sister. On one occasion he fastened her ankle to the inside of her crib to keep her in place. He assures me that the very weak string would have easily snapped if stressed and was too short to be of any danger. He also claims this one treatment did the trick but I think she outgrew it as expected. However, I believe that it's better to protect your kids by reducing the dangers in the ways that are presented below.

Everything is a matter of degree. If sleepwalking episodes are infrequent or relatively benign, such as raiding the refrigerator, mention it to your family doctor, who will put it on the radar screen for further monitoring. However, if they do occur often, and particularly if the sleepwalker leaves the house, or is injuring himself or herself or injuring other people, by all means talk to your doctor or a sleep specialist.

In a few instances, sleepwalking has been linked to violent behavior, something that also seems to happen in conjunction with an uncommon condition called REM behavior disorder, which will be explained later in this chapter. Shows of unconscious violence should immediately be subject to medical treatment.

An Arizona man was arrested for stabbing his wife 44 times and drowning her. Using parasomnia as a mitigating factor, he was acquitted on the grounds of temporary insanity. However, this defense has failed in many other cases. The take-home lesson is if the behavior is potentially dangerous or bizarre, don't wait to talk to your doctor.

WHAT CAN BE DONE TO PREVENT AROUSAL DISORDERS?

The first step in preventing arousal disorders is to become aware of things that can cause these disorders to grow worse.

Sleep terror disorder and sleepwalking seem to occur more often in association with fever, sleep deprivation (lack of sleep), and medication such as thioridazine, fluphenazine, perphenazine, and desipramine.

Sleepwalking disorder may result from a hereditary or familial tendency. Episodes may also occur in response to an internal or external signal (such as a full bladder or loud noise).

Some preventive measures include the following:

- Prepare for the best sleep possible by having a defined calming bedtime ritual. (Stress can trigger sleepwalking, and some people meditate, or do yoga or relaxation exercises.)
- Get plenty of rest, since being overtired can trigger sleepwalking.
- Calm down before bedtime.
- Remove sharp furniture that could be dangerous from the bedroom.
- Sleep on the ground floor if you are prone to wandering.
- Make it difficult to open windows by locking them and adding heavy drapes or doors. To foil advanced escape behavior, install alarms at all exits.

- Remove delicate furniture, electronic equipment, and mirrors from bedroom.

PROFESSIONAL TREATMENT OPTIONS

- Hypnosis has been effective with both children and adults.

If there has been dangerous or complicated behavior such as leaving the house, consider doing the following:

- Consult a psychiatrist to establish and treat any mental health issues.
- Get a thorough physical examination and have a sleep specialist review your current medications.

Medications called benzodiazepines, such as diazepam or lorazepam, can be used to treat arousal disorders when there is a danger to the sleeper or others. It is presumed that these medications convert the on-off switch to a more gentle "dimmer" type although the exact mechanism of how they work is not known. We do know that benzodiazepines affect the timing, quality, and quantity of sleep stages.

Sleep-Wake Transition Disorders

The second major category of parasomnias are those that occur during the transition from wakefulness to sleep, in the transition from sleep to wakefulness, or less frequently during the transition from one sleep stage to another. Examples include:

Sleep starts. These are very familiar to many of us—and to our bed partners. We are snatched back from our journey into sleep with a startled movement and perhaps a shout.

Sleep talking. Also quite common, this behavior is usually incoherent or amusing, and sometimes disturbing, to the listener.

Nocturnal leg cramps. These are generally benign but can be annoying. Fortunately they are not very common. They are also different from restless legs syndrome (see Chapter 9). Medically, the primary concern is that you may suffer from a vascular disease that doesn't permit enough blood to get to the muscles. A simple Doppler exam can establish blood flow. Mild analgesics, quinine, massages, and warm baths can also be helpful.

Rhythmic movement disorder. This can be quite disturbing to witness. Usually associated with boys ages six months to four years, it takes the form of several characteristic movements including head banging, head rolling, body rocking and body rolling, beginning just before sleep onset and continuing into light sleep. The episodes usually end when the person is disturbed or spoken to.

These children are often developmentally, behaviorally, and medically normal; the behavior rarely results in physical injury, and they usually outgrow it.

For adults who have movement disorders, treatment is sometimes needed if the movement delays the onset of sleep and leaves the patient excessively tired. Once again, the quality of life is key.

If cognitive or behavioral therapy fails, mild hypnotics, such as Ambien, or benzodiazepine can be used by adults for many muscle-movement disorders.

REM Sleep Parasomnias

You will recall from Chapter 2 that REM sleep is vital not only for psychological health but because it probably plays a central role in physical health as well. As I put it then, "REM sleep is a riot of electrical impulses so intense that if it happened when you were awake, you wouldn't be able to function." Atonia, the deactivation of your muscles except for those involved in keeping your heart beating and your lungs breathing, is a key mechanism of REM sleep because it keeps you in one place while your brain circuits are firing at peak levels.

The most common of REM sleep parasomnias are nightmares, dreams so frightening that they often wake us up. Almost every child hears the reassuring words "It's only a dream" at one time or another as they wake up "just in time."

We know from sleep studies that nightmares differ substantially from night terrors. Unlike terrors, which typically occur early in the night's sleep, nightmares usually take place in the second half. The effects on the body are different as well. For example, the heartbeat isn't explosively elevated the way it is in night terrors. Also, the dream content is usually fresh in the sleeper's mind.

In many adults, nightmares appear related simply to daytime stress or experience. Nightmares also seem to be linked to an increase in

REM sleep following a period of REM deficit caused by stress, use of certain drugs, including antidepressants and alcohol, or other causes. Such periods of catch-up sleep are known as sleep rebound, or REM rebound. Sleep debt, like all debts, has a payback, although you never truly zero out that debt.

If you experience recurring nightmares, treatment might include:

- Counseling on how to avoid recognizable sources of stress
- Psychotherapy
- Strict adherence to a program of sleep hygiene

If nightmares are ruining your life, proper medical treatment is a must, including extensive testing of your blood, and a complete physical examination. Medication can be used to suppress nightmares, although it may also suppress REM sleep, which is not always a good thing. Such a course of therapy should only be undertaken after testing and review by a sleep specialist.

Sleep paralysis. This is related to muscle atonia and can occur at times other than REM sleep. When it occurs in a state near to waking, the patient will become aware of the paralysis, which is disturbing, although it is otherwise harmless. One of those sleep-state switches may be temporarily out of whack, which happens to many of us from time to time, or it may be an isolated hereditary disorder that you can learn to live with.

However, when sleep paralysis is accompanied by other symptoms, such as excessive daytime sleepiness, cataplexy, vivid dreaming or hypnagogic hallucinations, it is associated with narcolepsy, which you read about in Chapter 8.

REM SLEEP BEHAVIOR DISORDER (REM BD)

This is an important one, because it contains the potential for violence, and damage to people and property. It occurs in an estimated 0.5 percent of the population.

I explained in Chapter 2 that atonia is important because if your muscles were functioning during the intense electrical activity in your brain that ignites dreaming, you might run through the wall. REM sleep behavior disorder is a state in which this protection is lost and dream content actually comes to life: The patient acts out his or her dreams.

This can be harmless, depending on the dream. Driving or fishing are benign. Being chased is more problematic—you have the potential for kicking a bed partner or tripping over the furniture if you make it out of bed. Fighting is worse, because the person you punch or choke may be a member of your family.

When a patient comes to us with complaints that indicate REM sleep behavior disorder, we look for specific characteristics to help make a differential diagnosis. For example, abnormal REM behavior is often connected to very serious neuropathology. At least one-third of patients who experience REM BD have a history of conditions such as dementia, subarachnoid hemorrhage, stroke, Parkinson's disease, multiple sclerosis, and Guillain-Barré syndrome.

Another possible association is between abnormal REM behavior and post-traumatic stress disorder. I am particularly sensitive to this one, since in New York City, we have a very large contingent of police and firefighters who have been on a state of high alert since 9/11.

A common precursor of REM BD is alcoholism. Because alcohol is a REM-suppressing substance, patients with a history of alcoholism can start to exhibit REM BD after they stop drinking, sometimes years later.

However, the majority of cases are idiopathic.

More men than women suffer from REM sleep disorders, and it is most frequent after the age of 60.

TREATMENT

The various medical conditions that underlie many cases of REM BD must be treated. If anxiety or post-traumatic stress are found to be factors, cognitive therapy and behavioral therapy might help. However, because of the severe nature of REM BD, chemical treatment must often be used.

Most cases respond to the benzodiazepine clonazepam, which is a sedative. This is an "off label" use of the drug, which suppresses both the violent behavior and the vivid recall of the related dreams that can produce continued anxiety during the day.

Another drug, Desipramine, an antidepressant, is also used "off label," to treat REM BD and is successful in some cases. And by all means, take precautions against injury.

Other Parasomnias

Teeth grinding (also known as bruxism), bed-wetting, and primary snoring are other examples of parasomnia.

In addition, there are other conditions that are easily confused with parasomnias, but which are not. These include:

- Anxiety disorders
- Panic disorders
- Sleep apnea arousals
- Geriatric sleep disorder (such as sundowning—confusing night and day)
- Epilepsy

Sex and Violence in Sleep

Sexual aggression in sleep and violence in sleep are real. They have substantial implications for the way people live, not only as a matter of medical health but as a matter of law.

VIOLENCE IN SLEEP

Researchers at Stanford University described the case of the father of a three-month-old boy who threw the child out a third-story window and then went rushing out into the street.

Fortunately the child landed on a canopy and survived with just a few scratches. However, the father was arrested for attempted murder and spent three months in jail with no memory of the incident. His lawyer secured a sleep study that produced some remarkable information.

The father had been a sleepwalker since the age of six. As a boy, the father had had frequent sleepwalking events and confusional arousals almost every night.

It also happened that in the period before the incident, an earthquake had destroyed their home, and the family slept through the aftershocks for two weeks in the stressful environment of a tent, with the lullaby of earth tremors. After extensive medical, psychiatric, and sleep study evaluations, the courts accepted a conclusion that the event was related to sleepwalking, and that medical care was needed. The experts felt that during the episode the father had sensed an immediate danger to his child and took an action that in his dream state was really an attempt to save the boy. The charges were dropped.

In another reported case, the wife of a 57-year-old man woke up at 2 A.M. to find herself being strangled. She only realized it was her husband when she heard him shouting, "I will kill you, you bastard." She got away from him while he continued to scream and beat the mattress. She pleaded with him to stop but he didn't respond. After a few minutes he fell asleep, and when he reawakened he had no memory of the episode. While she never reported it to the police, from then on she slept in a different bedroom with the door locked.

When he was evaluated, it turned out he had displayed abnormal sleep behavior for about five years, including making shouting noises and movements that occasionally bruised his wife. He was an enthusiastic golfer and would dream about the game. These dreams were acted out. The behavior was aggravated by drinking.

Shortly before the choking incident, there had been a burglary in the neighborhood. During the day he had expressed concern for his family's safety and he had had several dreams about confronting the burglars.

In both cases, there was a long delay between the occurrence of sleep-related symptoms and their being reported. As should be clear by now from reading this book, patients and their bed partners may be reticent about seeking help for abnormal behavior. If it is not violent, and this was true in both cases for a considerable amount of time, the bed partner faces a double burden—first convincing the person that his behavior during sleep is strange, and second, overcoming shame and embarrassment about revealing such behavior to an outsider.

While violence in sleep has been successfully used as a defense in courts of law, it is an intricate one to make. The hurdles are high. It would be very difficult to argue if it weren't true.

The criteria listed below are endorsed by the American Academy of Sleep Medicine as appropriate for a legal defense based on violence in sleep. However, they are also a useful list of indicators that might point to potential disturbances in "normal" homes. A comprehensive medical history must include:

- Detailed description of the event and the degree of amnesia
- History of current, past, or family sleep disorders
- Current, past, or family medical record
- Social habits
- Drug/medication/alcohol intake
- Employment records and difficulties potentially related to sleep disorders

- Determination of the frequency of violence and its stereotypic nature
- Description of prior events
- Timing of event during sleep-wake cycle
- Frequency of events over time
- Age at onset and associated life events/traumas
- Degree of amnesia noted
- Attitude of subject when fully awake after the event
- Attitude after previous sleep-related disturbances (if reported)
- Association of the abnormal behavior with daytime activities such as:
  a. Stress
  b. Sleep deprivation
  c. Drug/alcohol intake
  d. Febrile illness
  e. Life events

Thankfully, few cases will be serious enough to make it as far as the courts. However, 2 percent of Americans display symptoms of this behavior, there is grave potential for life, limb, and property just based on the arithmetic. If you suspect that your bed partner is displaying abnormal sleep behavior and is under inordinate levels of stress, I urge you to seek medical help.

SEXUAL AGGRESSION DURING SLEEP

This is a variation of sleep violence that is, if anything, more difficult to face than other forms of violence. Patients and their partners are ashamed and reluctant to report this behavior because it is a window into the murkier parts of their personality. Researchers have collected cases that include undressing of the partner, fondling, forced intercourse, and masturbation with no consciousness of the event. Moreover, the objects of this behavior have included not only adult partners but children of the same and opposite sex.

As with other violent sleep episodes, the behavior may be at diametric odds with the waking personality and conduct of the individual. This Dr. Jekyll and Mr. Hyde quality can put an unbearable burden on any marriage or relationship. A partner awakened by this person's alarming activity may wonder, "What kind of person is this *really?* Do I know [him or her]?"

Those are questions that are hard to answer in the best of relationships.

The symptoms ought to be self-evident, and if there is reason to suspect that this parasomnia is present, by all means seek professional help as you would with any other case of violence. The underlying conditions are too complex to deal with on your own.

WHAT CAN BE DONE?

In the short term, during diagnosis and treatment, you and your bed partner can take precautions:

- Sleep in separate beds or bedrooms.
- The subject could sleep in a sleeping bag with zipper fully zipped to impede hand movement and the ability to move generally.
- You might take many of the precautions listed earlier for sleep-walking, again always using common sense and putting safety for both patient and partner or others in the household at the top of the list.

Pharmacological Treatment

- Antiepileptic medication if parasomnia is related to seizure
- Clonazepam for REM sleep behavior disorder
- Benzodiazepines (diazepam, clonazepam, temazepam) for non-REM sleep parasomnia
  All of the above are potentially dangerous medications with significant side effects even at low doses.

TESTING FOR PARASOMNIAS

No specific testing is necessary for parasomnias especially if episodes are infrequent and not associated with injury or dangerous behavior. Discuss the symptoms with your doctor and if he or she suspects a medical or psychiatric condition, further testing may be necessary.

A sleep study may be necessary if there is uncertainty about the diagnosis, if there are unexplained disruptive nighttime or daytime symptoms, or if an additional sleep disorder is suspected.

Most children outgrow parasomnias. Parasomnias starting in adulthood tend to be chronic and may become a periodic problem for life.

It must be pointed out that not all parasomnia activity is a threat either to the sleeper or the bed partner. Some sleepwalking, talking, and movement can be annoying and occasionally entertaining to onlookers. For many somnambulists, the worst that happens is that they wake up to find empty ice cream containers on the kitchen table and maybe gain a bit of weight. With help in a healthy marriage or domestic partnership, a couple will work out a way of dealing with the habits of one.

For example, I am an enthusiastic golfer and I very occasionally practice it in my sleep. My wife sleeps to my right and I swing to my left. I don't yell "Fore" and I haven't hit her yet.

"WHAT'S THE MATTER WITH KIDS TODAY?"

Does your child snore loudly?

Is your child overweight and does he or she have large tonsils?

In addition to the above, does your child have allergic nasal congestion?

Does your child have to be awakened on most mornings?

During the day does your child seem overtired, cranky, irritable, aggressive, overemotional, hyperactive, or to have trouble thinking, and do you hear complaints from teachers?

When you drive with your child in the car, does he or she fall asleep almost every time?

Does your child "crash" much earlier than usual on some nights?

The more questions you answer "yes" to, the greater the chances are the child has a sleep problem, and you ought to tell your doctor about it.

What's the matter with kids today? Maybe they're not getting enough sleep, or the right kind of sleep.

- Infants get 12.7 hours, when experts recommend that from ages 3 to 11 months they should get 14 to 15 hours.
- Toddlers get 11.7 hours, when 12 to 14 hours are recommended for children aged 1 to 3 years.
- Preschoolers get 10.4 hours, while it's recommended that children 3–5 years of age should average 11 to 13 hours.
- School-age children (first through fifth grades) get 9.5 hours, but experts recommend 10 to 11 hours.

Source: 2004 Sleep in America poll, the first nationwide survey on the sleep habits of children and their parents, conducted by the National Sleep Foundation.

The conventional wisdom about "early to bed and early to rise" is based on the assumption that children's sleeping habits are mostly a matter of parental example, supervision, and values. Starting with infancy, children have been subject to many rules and rituals, some of which directly contradict one another. These involve, among other things, feeding times, bathing, rocking and cuddling, lullabies, stories and prayers, night-lights, mobiles hovering over them, swaddling, not sleeping on their stomachs, pillows, no pillows, comforting when they cry, not comforting them when they cry, use of juice bottles, no juice bottles, taking them to bed with Mom and Dad (or *not*), and so on.

At each developmental stage new rules take over, some of which are quite modern and some of which go back generations. The one consistent theme throughout all these rules is that they are based primarily on the desire to raise healthy, happy children, and secondarily on their parents' desire to keep themselves from going crazy.

One example of how the parents' desire to buy peace at bedtime conflicts with the child's interests is the use of juice bottles at bedtime. Parents who let their children have juice bottles because it keeps them quiet until they fall asleep are a dentist's best friends because all that concentrated fruit sugar will rot those cute little baby teeth. Root canal for four-year-olds is not unheard-of among the juice-at-bedtime crowd.

The challenge of bedtime becomes harder to tackle as children get older and continue to develop minds of their own. While the invention of the electric light bulb has done more to change mankind's sleeping habits than any event since the discovery of fire, new uses of electricity represent a new threat to the sleep of each generation. Radio, telephones, television, computers, Internet—the parade of new appliances makes staying up a little longer at night a more attractive prospect than going to sleep. Twenty percent of *infants* now have televisions in their bedroom, a number that more than doubles by school age. When you consider that we recommend that adults not have televisions in their bedrooms, think about the effects the tube will have on children's sleep and developing brains.

Huge numbers of preschool and school-age children drink beverages that contain caffeine, and they get less sleep than other children, according to the National Sleep Foundation poll cited above. When you add up the amount of caffeine in the soft drinks and chocolate that children consume, the numbers may be alarming. Often the sleep diary helps uncover a weekly excess of caffeine that would otherwise be missed.

It takes strong parents to stand firm in the face of relentless arguments by their children. That's where parental example, supervision, and values come into play. Parents need to be disciplined in how we deal with the children in their evening waking hours as well as at their bedtimes. We also need to set an example. When you're a child, staying up late always looks like more fun than going to bed. We have to show them that bedtime is important for us, too. The stronger the foundation we lay early in life of modeling bedtime as a secure, warm, and happy time, the greater the likelihood that our children will have good associations with it throughout their lives. Except, occasionally, for my own kids.

In addition to the scientific development mentioned above, there's another side of science and technology at work here, and that is the ability it has now given us to appreciate the effects of poor sleep on our children. We now can use—and we need to—the most current scientific discoveries about sleep to reinforce the more sensible rules our parents and grandparents taught us and to do away with the ones that don't make sense. However, we must also be alert to the possibility that our children's sleep problems are based on something other than the absence of routine and parental discipline. Children can be afflicted with many physical ailments that adults are susceptible to, as well as some that are more prevalent at an early age, and the need for treatment is just as urgent.

Sunrise, Sunset

One message scientific evidence sends is that we have to do more to ensure respect for the rhythms that evolved in us in response to the movement of the earth around the sun.

We can see this quite vividly in the experience of infants who are kept for considerable amounts of time in the hospital. It was common practice in many nurseries to keep bright lights on all the time. This made it easier for round-the-clock staff to do their jobs, but it's not good for the children. When infants are subject to cycles of bright and dim light, they have been shown to sleep longer, feed earlier, and grow better than those who get nonstop bright light.

This distinction is quite logical. Animal research has shown that the biological clock (its technical name is the suprachiasmatic nucleus, or SCN—discussed in Chapter 2) starts to work during the middle and latter stages of gestation—the period that is cut short by premature birth. If the same pattern of SCN development holds for human infants as for animals, which is a good bet, this critical phase of neurological development is at risk of being disrupted by bright lights. In recognition of these scientific discoveries, new regulations for neonatal wards have been written ordering that lighting in the nurseries be adjusted to more closely mimic natural lighting cycles.

The march of scientific knowledge has also drastically changed other ways we treat our children during pregnancy and beyond. For example, two generations ago, women smoked and drank routinely during pregnancy. Now we know that smoking causes low birth weight, and that drinking during pregnancy causes fetal alcohol syndrome. A generation ago, there was no data to support the idea that secondhand smoke is dangerous to children or anyone else. Now we know that it causes many problems in people of all ages, from allergies to increased risk of heart attacks and strokes.

So much has been discovered and written about the effects of prenatal and neonatal care on our children over the past generation that attentive parents devote a great deal of time and family resources trying to create "perfect" children, as if there were any such thing. For all the care that moms and dads devote to giving up cigarettes, cutting down on drinking, and eating right, however, much less attention is given to sleep issues. And of course, among parents who are less attentive to these basics, sleep is even more neglected. Among parents of all classes, their children's bedtime habits are often more a matter of convenience than of long-term health.

Dangers of Suppressing REM Sleep

Studies of young animals have shown that suppressing REM sleep can alter behavior, physical development, and biochemistry in ways that affect the animals throughout their lives.

When newborn rats don't get enough REM sleep, it changes their breathing patterns, their metabolism, the concentration of neurotransmitters in different parts of the brain, and the receptors for those neurotransmitters. These changes are lifelong, which indicates that disruption of infants' sleep causes permanent miswiring of the brain.

People are animals, too. Why should it be any different for small children than for other small mammals?

Infant brains are highly "plastic," which means that they grow in response to different kinds of stimulation. Brain development is "activity dependent." To get the brain to function the way it's supposed to, it needs to experience the right kind of stimulation. For example, the ability to see depends on exposure to light, objects, and so forth. Studies suggest that maternal and paternal contact is important for emotional development. The "lessons learned" by the brain are then consolidated during REM sleep.

Newborn children sleep an average of 16 out of 24 hours and spend the majority of their sleeping time in REM sleep. That REM sleep is necessary—their brains have to build a foundation for a lifetime of learning in the first six months of life. If that 80-20 percent balance of REM and non-REM sleep is disrupted by being awake when they should be asleep, the ripples will be felt throughout the growing infant's life. The pain of colic, the discomfort of a wet diaper, loud noises—these and many more uncomfortable sensory stimuli can disturb the brain when it should be doing other things. After the age of six months, they sleep somewhat less and that sleep is distributed slightly differently, with most of their sleep being at night and the rest in the form of daytime naps.

The Tragedy of SIDS

Despite a dramatic decline in deaths related to sudden infant death syndrome (SIDS), also known as crib death, mainly due to worldwide educational campaigns, SIDS remains a major cause of sudden death in African Americans. SIDS death rates are more than twice as high among African Americans as those of other racial groups, although recent research is pointing to at least some indication that there is a genetic component to SIDS for all groups.

The following key measures are recommended for the care of infants. Please share the pertinent recommendations with everyone you know who cares for an infant.

Also, during pregnancy, do not smoke or drink alcohol. And, regular prenatal checkups for mothers and infants are essential.

- Always place infants on their backs at bedtime and naptime.
- Remove pillows and soft toys from the crib.
- Make sure the infant's head and face aren't covered by the blanket.
- Use a firm, tight-fitting mattress.
- Infants should not share beds with other infants or an adult.
- Dress infants comfortably but do not allow them to become overheated.
- Keep the room temperature comfortable, as for adults.
- Keep a smoke-free environment around infants.
- Call a physician immediately if the infant is ill.
- Breast feeding may offer protection against SIDS.
- Putting the infant to sleep with a pacifier may offer some protection.

Sleep-Disordered Breathing and Sleep Apnea among Children

We can't blame all our children's sleep problems on the harnessing of electricity and the ways we use it. The most serious sleep problems that children, like older people, face are sleep-disordered breathing and sleep apnea.

As with adults, the incidence of this condition can partially be attributed to that modern plague of overweight. We are continually reminded that kids don't get enough exercise. They eat the wrong food and they eat too much food. An estimated 13 percent of children aged 6 to 11, and 14 percent of adolescents aged 12 to 19 are overweight. As with their elders, this puts them at risk not only for heart disease, type 2 diabetes, and high blood pressure but for sleep apnea as well.

Unlike their elders, however, children are still growing, and that makes sleep apnea even more ominous for them than it is for grown-ups. For a snoring 40-year-old, a good night's sleep is necessary for restoring and maintaining a mature body and mind. But for a child, whose body and mind are still growing, the effects of sleep apnea are likely to influence the kind of person the child will become, and not for the better.

The higher immediate risks of sleep disorders to children's health may also be behavioral and psychological rather than physical. In one study, children suspected of having sleep-disordered breathing scored significantly worse than a control group on all categories in the Pediatric Quality of Life Inventory, which records parents' perceptions about their children, and the Children's Depression Inventory, which the children fill out themselves.

Attention-Deficit/Hyperactivity Disorder

Like many fathers may age, I have been raised by my children on a regular diet of *The Simpsons.* Bart, the reigning poster child of attention-deficit/hyperactivity disorder (ADHD), is treated in one episode with "Focusin," a spoof of Ritalin, a stimulant.

Doctors prescribe Ritalin for ADHD because it usually works. Teachers and parents alike welcome the transformation. But in some cases the use of a stimulant to treat ADHD symptoms raises serious questions. We may be using a drug to treat a symptom without thoroughly considering other underlying medical conditions. Inattention in class is not only a symptom of ADHD. It is also associated with excessive daytime sleepiness, which of course is a symptom of any number of sleep disorders, including apnea, snoring, and narcolepsy.

Poor Sleep and ADHD?

Even a single night's inadequate sleep causes mood changes, the inability to focus and concentrate, and can lead to impulsive behavior. Chronic poor sleep aggravates these problems. These symptoms can easily be mistaken for symptoms of ADHD. To appreciate the similarity, you have only to look at the criteria for diagnosing ADHD. The following are the criteria for inattentiveness set forth by the American Psychiatric Association's *Diagnostic and Statistical Manual of Mental Disorders* revised fourth edition. (There are also symptoms for hyperactivity and impulsiveness, although we have chosen not to list them.) A child must exhibit six or more symptoms of inattention for at least six months to "a degree that is not consistent with the normal expected behavior for the person's age." Moreover, the symptoms must be observed both at school and at home (for adults it can be work and home).

a. Often fails to give close attention to details or makes careless mistakes in schoolwork, work, or other activities
b. Often has difficulty sustaining attention in tasks or play activities
c. Often does not seem to listen when spoken to directly
d. Often does not follow through on instructions and fails to finish schoolwork, chores, or duties in the workplace (not due to oppositional behavior or failure to understand instructions)
e. Often has difficulty organizing tasks and activities
f. Often avoids, dislikes, or is reluctant to engage in tasks that require sustained mental effort, such as schoolwork or homework
g. Often loses things necessary for tasks or activities, such as toys, school assignments, pencils, books, or tools
h. Is often easily distracted by things around him or her
i. Is often forgetful in daily activities

Years ago, a child with these symptoms might have been labeled a "cutup" or as "going through a phase" or "slow learner." If it went on for too long, however, the child might end up branded an underachiever or become a school dropout. Today, at least, such children get some medical attention—with the diagnosis of ADHD. Since a diagnosis of ADHD must encompass behavior at school as well as at home, we have done a wonderful job of educating teachers and school nurses about symptoms and enlisting them as partners in helping these children.

The question is whether it is the right kind of medical attention. Is every prescription for Ritalin the right therapy? When it comes to ADHD, doctors are now focusing on new evidence that helps them move beyond the "no child left unprescribed" era.

In fact, this list of symptoms of inattentiveness is very similar to the list of symptoms seen in children with obstructive sleep apnea, and untreated sleep apnea in children is associated with poor performance in school and at home. But ADHD has become the default diagnosis. Children who come to the sleep lab with severe sleep apnea generally have airways that are blocked by enlarged tonsils and/or adenoids. The associated symptoms of sleepiness, inattentiveness, and poor school performance make perfect sense. Their nighttime problems are affecting their daytime behavior.

I have seen several patients in their early 20s who were treated for ADHD for many years and who, when studied, turned out to have moderate to severe sleep apnea. They certainly may have had two separate conditions but what if they hadn't? Their lives might have been very different if they had been treated for their sleep-disordered breathing rather than for ADHD.

Complicating the picture still further is the fact that younger children deprived of sleep do not always show obvious signs of being tired, but rather become hyperactive and irritable. Many people speak glibly about the apparently paradoxical effect that Ritalin and other stimulants seem to have on young ADHD patients: It calms them down rather than speeds them up, in contrast to adults. This may be no paradox at all, and that in fact in many cases stimulants used to treat ADHD may be waking tired children. The fact is that we don't really know what "normal" is for every child.

Children with sleep apnea who receive Ritalin seem to improve, but why and what exactly are we treating? Children who snore regularly should be screened by their doctor for sleep apnea if they have other nighttime symptoms, such as restless sleep, labored breathing or sweating, or daytime symptoms with a diagnosis of ADHD (either the inattentive or hyperactive variety).

The Snoring Connection

Eight percent of children in the general population snore. Thirty-three percent of those diagnosed with ADHD snore. Is there a connection?

Boys eight years old and younger who have habitual snoring are 4.3 times more likely to have ADHD than boys who do not snore. Again, is there a connection?

A study published in the journal *Pediatrics* in March 2003 found that about one-quarter of five- to seven-year-old children with mild symp-

Breathing Free

As with grown-ups, the real basis for obstructive breathing in children may be physical. It may be allergies. It may be the shape of the jaw. Very often it is the tonsils, adenoids, or swollen tissue from upper-airway allergies.

There was a time was when removing a child's tonsils was a common medical procedure. Kids loved it because they were forced to eat nothing but ice cream for several days. This operation fell out of favor as a routine procedure because as part of the lymph system, tonsils were thought to play some role in fighting infection. Furthermore, there was a movement afoot to reduce unnecessary surgery. So for another generation, kids put up with tonsillitis and throat infections.

However, having your tonsils out may be "in" again. Adeno-tonsillectomy—removal of adenoids and tonsils—is estimated to be effective in 95 percent of children who snore or have sleep apnea. Furthermore, it may be a boon for overall health. The annual medical bills for children with obstructive sleep apnea fell by nearly a third after adenotonsillectomy, according to a study done in Israel. Specific physiologic effects include the reversal of one of the most troubling effects of apnea—the suppression of growth hormone secretion. According to the Israeli study, six months after surgery children showed higher concentrations of the crucial hormones. Measures of weight, height, and the ratio of fat to body weight all showed considerable improvement.

The Nose Knows

One medical specialty that has common cause with sleep medicine is allergy and immunology, and for good reason. Pediatric allergists particularly are our invaluable allies in helping young patients. As a pulmonologist—a breathing specialist—I particularly appreciate this common purpose.

Paul Ehrlich, long one of the top pediatric allergists in New York and certified in both allergy and pediatrics, cites the following factors in his lectures to students and other doctors:

- Disruption of nighttime sleep impairs daytime wakefulness, cognitive functioning, psychomotor speed and coordination, and mood.
- Children with perennial allergic rhinitis have *significant sleep disturbance*.
- In a study of 54 first graders with obstructive sleep apnea, 24 of them underwent tonsillectomy and adenoidectomy. The mean grades of treated students during the second grade *increased significantly*. No academic improvement occurred in the untreated group.
- The presence of nasal congestion associated with allergic rhinitis is a risk factor for *obstructive sleep apnea*.
- A study of 39 children with habitual snoring found the frequency of obstructive sleep apnea was 50 percent greater for allergic than nonallergic subjects.
- A survey of 400 parents with allergic and nonallergic children found that allergic children were significantly *more withdrawn and drowsy*.

Furthermore, inflammation and fluid in the eustachian tubes, the tubes that go from the nasopharynx to the middle ear, a common problem in allergic rhinitis, was found to be strongly related to *inattentiveness* and overtalkativeness.

Treating allergic rhinitis is one of the simplest, and to me, most effective ways of treating sleep disorders. However, not all treatments are alike. For example, Benadryl, an over-the-counter antihistamine (discussed in Chapter 7), is an effective allergy drug; it is still recommended by pediatricians and allergists even though there are several generations of new treatments. However, because it is a sedative, it may make your child even sleepier at school. Any drug that comes with a warning not to drive or operate heavy machinery can't be good for attentiveness at school. Claritin, a second generation nonsedating antihistamine, is also available over the counter. Other nonsedating allergy drugs, such as Singulair, are by prescription.

A well-cleaned bedroom is particularly important for a child with nasal allergies, and an air filtration device is also recommended.

If your child has persistent nasal and other allergies, you would be well advised to consult with a pediatric allergist who can test for seasonal, dietary, and environmental allergies and recommend a comprehensive course of treatment, possibly including allergy shots.

Leg Movements and ADHD

A study of children with ADHD and periodic limb movement disorders (PLMD) found that in many cases in which PMLD was treated with L-dopa (also called levodopa), the symptoms of ADHD improved. L-dopa is traditionally used to treat Parkinson's disease and limb movement disorders but was not previously known to have an effect on symptoms of ADHD. But doctors have reported in recent years improvement in most of the cases of ADHD in which children were treated with L-dopa, especially in the symptoms connected with their behavior, mental acuity, attention spans, and memory. Researchers are not certain why levodopa impacts on the children's ADHD symptoms; however, they hypothesize that a common link—a dopaminergic deficiency in the brain—causes both the sleep disorders and the ADHD.

The parents of children with ADHD and PLMD have a higher incidence of restless legs syndrome than other parents, suggesting a hereditary link. Heredity should be considered a factor in most sleep disorders. Researchers in London who studied 2,000 sets of female twins found that 50 percent of the variation in sleep disorders could be traced to genetics, particularly with obstructive sleep apnea and limb movement disorders.

Narcolepsy

You are now familiar with narcolepsy, having read Chapter 8. One big difference between pediatric narcolepsy and adult narcolepsy is that excessive daytime sleepiness is the primary symptom for children rather than cataplexy.

Paranormal Behavior—Parasomnia

No, there's nothing supernatural about it. Your child isn't suddenly seized by something out of *Ghostbusters* or channeling a past life. But, as discussed in Chapter 11, he or she might appear that way. Night terrors, incoherent babbling, urinating in bed, and other abnormal behaviors are generally not physically damaging in and of themselves, but they can be disruptive to the family, demoralizing to the child, and potentially dangerous to others and to property as well as to the child.

Many other childhood sleep disorders, such as somnambulism, talking while asleep, and rocking back and forth are actually types of parasomnia. They are more common among children than among adults, and children tend to outgrow them before they hit their teens. Parents may notice an increase in frequency or intensity when the child is sick, taking certain medications, or experiencing stress.

The following are the major categories of parasomnia to watch for.

DISORIENTED AROUSALS

Disoriented arousals are more common among children than among adults. They may begin with yelling or crying and violently moving in bed. Your child will seem to be alert and upset, but your efforts to comfort him or her will probably be futile. Still, it can be upsetting to confront a beloved child who is in the midst of one of these episodes, which can last up to half an hour, after which the sleeper may wake up and then go back to sleep.

SLEEPWALKING

Sleepwalking is the stuff of cartoons and movies, but it is a real phenomenon. The sleepwalker's vision and ability to perceive danger appear to operate, although there are reports of injury. The normal precautions for childproofing a room—no sharp edges, gates at the top of the stairs, floors clear of toys at bedtime, and intercoms to monitor the noise of the child's movements are advised. Episodes can last from minutes to an hour.

NIGHT/SLEEP TERRORS

As I mentioned in Chapter 11, this was my specialty as a child. Night terrors are very different from nightmares, which are associated with REM or dream sleep. Night terrors are frightening, but they don't usually have a story.

Terrors typically begin with a bloodcurdling scream, increased heart and breathing rates, sweating, and a frightened expression and last from one to several minutes. The child will probably not remember the episode, although the rest of the family might.

Sleep Tips for Your School-Age Children

1. Introduce healthy sleep habits as an overall program of disease prevention, including regular checkups, exercise, and diet.
2. Emphasize the need for a regular and consistent sleep schedule and bedtime routine.
3. The child's bedroom should be dark, cool, and quiet. TVs and computers should be off and out of the bedroom.
4. Avoid drinks and sweets that contain caffeine.
5. Watch for signs of chronic difficulty sleeping, loud snoring, difficulty breathing, unusual nighttime awakenings, and frequent daytime sleepiness.

A Web site of the National Sleep Foundation—www .sleepforkids.org—advises that you talk to your doctor if you observe any of the following:

- A newborn or infant who is extremely and consistently fussy
- A child having problems breathing or whose breathing is noisy (This applies at all times, not just while the child is asleep.)
- A child snoring, especially if the snoring is loud
- Unusual nighttime awakenings
- Difficulty falling asleep and maintaining sleep, especially if you see daytime sleepiness and/or behavioral problems

The "Vast Wasteland"

Years ago when a television executive described TV as "a vast wasteland," he was commenting on the content of the programs. While there is a tremendous amount of junk on TV still, the bigger problem is not what's on but how it is used, particularly by children and their parents. It has been called "the plug-in drug." Parents use it as an electronic babysitter and as a consequence, many kids do watch too much.

Television has been proven convincingly to affect brain development in ways that make it harder for children to concentrate, to learn, and to interact with other people. Slumping in front of the TV not only makes their brains lazy, however, but it also makes their bodies lazy. Moreover, they see commercials for fast food and candy and then demand that their parents buy it for them. They are likely to "graze" on snack foods while they watch.

This is pertinent for sleep medicine in several ways. First, the fattening of American children puts them at greater risk for snoring and sleep apnea at younger ages, as well as the accompanying medical conditions such as high blood pressure, diabetes, and heart disease.

Second, watching TV late in the evening interferes with the discipline of a routine that is crucial for good sleep hygiene. Watching an exciting action show or a sitcom just before bed is likely to wire kids up, not slow them down.

Third, more and more children have televisions in their bedrooms. This is bad when grown-ups do it. It's worse for children. And if they fall asleep with the TV on, the sound and light will interfere with the depth and quality of sleep they need for brain and body growth.

Finally, watching TV may affect brain wave activity in ways that will compromise the quality of sleep. There is a correlation between excessive TV watching and insomnia. Certain brain wave activity should take place only at the appropriate times during the sleep-wake cycle in order to get the most out of each. If the passive mental processes of TV watching cause parts of the brain to, in effect, go to sleep while our children are nominally awake, it stands to reason that it will affect the quality of their sleep later on. Just as sleep disturbance can lead to excessive daytime sleepiness, so it is likely that "waking disturbance" can result in excessive nighttime wakefulness.

Sleep diaries are very helpful in assuring that our children get the proper amount and quality of sleep. Often we are too busy to notice what they are doing or just not aware of things like drinking cola for lunch or eating a chocolate bar before bed. We have to make an effort to find these things out. In addition, patterns of watching late-night TV or surfing the Net will show up on a truthfully completed diary. As in other aspects of good parenting, this type of caring interaction often has the added value of being quality time. If the diary is filled out conscientiously with the child, it can be a form of companionship rather than a chore.

The pediatric sleep diary is located on pages 282–3.

Watching Over Our Children

We all have a responsibility to be concerned about and to watch over the welfare of our children. Pediatricians always strive to make us more aware of the disorders of the mind and body that can impact on a child's future. The information must get to those who spend the most time with our children, including, parents, teachers, and all caregivers.

In the past this vigilance has helped us identify and treat poor hygiene, inadequate nutrition, and conditions such as ADHD. We need to expand the range of what we are looking for, however. If we can work together we can start to define children's health in terms of a 24-hour day. For example, when we marvel at a week's worth of milestones achieved by a healthy child, we should remember that they needed about three days (72 hours) of healthy sleep to accomplish their goals. If daytime performance is a concern, we must include questions about nighttime behavior as part of the investigation. As should be clear by now, many sleep disorders may be present during the day and can appear like other daytime medical or behavioral disorders. Our common goal should be to treat all sleep disorders early and appropriately and to prevent them from occurring in the first place.

UNIQUE CHANGES—WOMEN AND SLEEP

Leah, a 70-year-old woman, recently widowed, came to my office complaining of insomnia. Her daughter Rebecca, who was with her, was very concerned about her mother, who had not slept well for 40 years—understandably since, among other things, she was a Holocaust survivor.

After a full examination and discussion I was convinced that Leah did indeed have insomnia; however, it was mild and chronic. Her complaint was not her daytime functioning or any physical or psychological problem but rather her expectations of and general thoughts about sleep. She was also in great physical shape for her age.

In fact, it was not the mother who gave me the greatest concern but rather Rebecca. In recounting the history, Rebecca described how she shared a house with her mom. She looked after her own seven children and her career as a principal. She calmly described a grueling schedule of home upkeep, custodial care, parenting, and self-preservation. Leah had had a tough life. She had many reasons to view the world of sleep as a lonely and unhappy place. Rebecca, on the other hand, was one of those "natural eagles" as a result of her ultra-multitasking. Like many women, including those in my own family, she took care of everyone else's needs before her own, and that took its silent toll. All that, and hormone flux, too.

Adding another layer of sometimes unpredictable and recurrent monthly hormone surge were three daughters stricken with severe premenstrual syndrome (the effects of PMS on mood and sleep are discussed later in this chapter). Rebecca went on to say, "As a teacher I would approach the problems of the day head-on with plenty of listening and then talking. The mother—and daughter—in me would always take over, however, and after a particularly bad day and third round, I would find myself up after midnight stressed and unable to sleep." By the time the weekend came around, Rebecca was exhausted and needed to catch up on missed sleep. She convinced her mother to come in for a sleep evaluation thinking to handle one issue at a time. As it turns out, the three generations in Rebecca's home exemplify sleep disorders common to women of all ages.

Not Created Exactly Equal

In general, sleep problems affect women more than men. More women have insomnia several times a week than men, and women are more likely to have daytime symptoms. A 1998 poll by the National Sleep Foundation revealed that women aged 30 through 60 averaged six hours and 41 minutes of sleep per night during the work week. As a result, they accumulate a huge sleep deficit. Remember that during the week when the clocks go forward by an hour in the spring and we are short *a single hour* of sleep, the accident rate goes up by 7 percent. Apply a somewhat larger deficit to the average woman, as defined by the 1998 study, and think of all the ways their lives may suffer—excessive daytime sleepiness, proneness to accidents, poor job performance, low energy. Older women are also more likely to report sleep problems over the prior 10 years more frequently than men.

Less well-documented is the possibility that disturbed sleep and sleepiness add to weight gain by discouraging physical activity and that depressed REM sleep encourages overeating. Apart from the blow to self-image from weight gain, it also exacerbates the tendency toward sleep apnea. It's a vicious downward spiral.

Natural Eagles

Part of the explanation for their sleep deficit is that many women live like eagles, either by choice or by necessity. They often don't have the luxury of settling into their natural circadian rhythm of lark or owl (discussed in detail in Chapter 4). They try to juggle home life, work, and an active social life at the expense of sleep. Complicate their lives with children, especially young ones, and a less-than-supportive partner and there's a good chance they will not be able to find the time to make up their sleep deficit on the weekend.

Aside from these external forces, another critical impediment to a good night's sleep is the internal fluctuation of hormones.

Women have not been studied carefully as a separate group in general and this is especially true for the age group beginning after menopause. There may be unique and permanent changes in sleep after menopause when estrogen and progesterone are no longer putting the body through its paces after 40 years or so of hard work. Postmenopausal women start to have sleep disturbances similar to those of men of the same age. In fact, the incidence of sleep apnea in women over the age of 50 increases steadily and approaches that of men.

CHANGE OF HEART

Research at our center, which we have presented recently at a national meeting, shows that postmenopausal women with obstructive sleep apnea syndrome have important EKG changes, which we refer to as QT interval prolongation. QT interval prolongation has been associated with heart arrhythmias and a higher risk for sudden death. Since this finding was not seen in premenopausal women, we hypothesized that the postmenopausal change in hormonal patterns, with the loss of estrogen protection, adds risk not only for apnea but for QT interval changes.

MEN HAVE IT EASY

We have to admit that women in many ways are more resilient and possibly the stronger of the two sexes. In between childhood and menopause, for example, are those uniquely female years of menstrual cycles, pregnancy, and menopause and the hormonal fluctuations that go with them. This is something that men just cannot identify with. The closest we can get is reading accounts in the sports pages of how anabolic steroids, which are derived from testosterone, have wrecked athletes' lives and the lives of those around them by contributing to outrageous mood swings and overaggressiveness both on the playing field and off.

Hormones and Moods

PMS has gotten a bad name. These initials are often cited by men and women as shorthand to disparage women's behavior. However, the behavior is part of a predictable hormone physiology that can affect sleep, among other things. The resulting sleep problems can account for some of the mood changes associated with PMS. We see similar mood changes in those who abuse anabolic steroids, as well as in patients, men and women, who receive hormones as part of treatment for certain cancers and in patients who have tumors that cause their adrenal glands to secrete extra cortisol, which is an essential steroid naturally produced by our body.

Fifty percent of women report that bloating by itself disturbs their sleep. Men don't bloat except when they are ill. Most women experience pain during their periods, which is not conducive to either a good night's sleep or a productive, active day. Men don't experience that level of regular abdominal cramping. Neither do most of us donate six pints of blood a year nor shed the lining of a major organ. One stereotype of men is that we have a low threshold for discomfort when we are ill. I confess that I am as bad as anyone in this regard, possibly because I am a doctor and I know all the things that could be wrong with me based on the symptoms. Complaints that routinely occur in women during their menstrual cycles are enough to keep men, including me, home from work and in bed. Yet women persevere.

WOMEN AND DEEP SLEEP

Deep sleep should comprise 15 to 20 percent of sleep during adulthood. Body tissues, which are worn out during the normal wear and tear of living, require deep sleep to repair themselves. This is recovery sleep, or beauty sleep, if you prefer, and women don't want less of it. Among other things, they have to rebuild the lining of their uterus.

Their bone marrow has to replace the blood cells they lose. Yet, they get 5 percent less deep sleep per month than men, which means their bodies have to do more work with less sleep.

Sleep disorders in women can be grouped according to the presence, absence, or fluctuations in sex hormones and the effect of those changes on the body and mind. In keeping with the concept of stressors discussed in Chapter 10, the wear and tear of these stressors affect the entire 24-hour day.

Sleep and the Menstrual Cycle

The average onset of premenstrual syndrome (PMS) is 26 years of age, and symptoms often become worse over time. The first few days of menstrual bleeding are the least restful—36 percent of women report unsatisfying sleep during their periods. Sleep is disturbed on average about 60 hours a month. (Again, I don't know what otherwise healthy men would do if their sleep were disturbed 60 hours a month. I don't know what *I* would do.) In the days after ovulation, women may find it difficult to fall asleep, possibly because progesterone levels are falling. As you will read in the section on pregnancy below, elevated progesterone levels early in pregnancy seem to be linked with stronger sleep tendency.

Insomnia and hypersomnia are among the most common effects of premenstrual syndrome (PMS) on sleep. Healthy sleepers spend 15–20 percent of their sleeping time in deep sleep, although, as mentioned earlier, women in general get less deep sleep than men. Women with PMS do far worse. They have all types of insomnia, and have reduced deep sleep all month long.

Premenstrual Dysphoric Disorder (PMDD)

Most doctors believe PMS and PMDD refer to the same clinical entity, but that is incorrect. PMS refers to the physical and mood symptoms that appear during the last one or two weeks of the menstrual cycle and disappear by the end of menses. PMDD is a diagnosis used by doctors to describe a specific set of mood symptoms that are also present the week before menses and remit a few days after the start of menses. Most women—75–85 percent—have cyclic menses symptoms, but only about 3–5 percent have symptoms so severe that they interfere with work, school, usual activities, or relationships.

PMS is defined more as physical symptoms such as bloating, weight gain, and breast tenderness, whereas PMDD has as part of its definition symptoms such as depressed mood, emotional volatility, irritability, decreased interest in usual activities, concentration difficulties, lack of energy, marked change in appetite, overeating or food cravings, feelings of being overwhelmed, and sleepiness or insomnia.

Charting the Changes

K.B. was a 21-year-old prelaw student who came to the sleep center complaining of insomnia. She had a history of "occasional" mild depression although she had never seen a psychologist or psychiatrist. An occasional Ambien did not help the insomnia, which seemed to come and go in synch with the feelings of low energy. As part of the workup she completed a one-month sleep diary and on review we noticed a pattern of insomnia and mood disturbance coinciding with a certain time of her menstrual period. Over the next several months she improved with a combination of cognitive and behavioral therapy along with Ambien taken for five to seven days as predicted by the previous month's sleep diary. In time she experienced fewer bad days during the month, slept better, and used less Ambien.

A day diary is a very useful tool to help make the diagnosis of PMS or PMDD. Charting symptoms day-by-day and correlating them with the general sleep diary or log is invaluable not only for the diagnosis of menses-related disorders but also for sleep disorders. Recall alone is not reliable, especially if the doctor visit is two to three weeks after the fact. The diary helps you see a pattern of daytime symptoms and makes the connection to the associated sleep disturbance more obvious.

(Refer to the general sleep diary on pages 280–81 in the back of the book.)

Treatment of Menstruation-Related Sleep Disorders

Generally, menstrual-related insomnia disappears a few days after menstruation ends. However, tension and irritability associated with menstruation may result in persistent sleep problems leading to chronic insomnia. Maintaining a regular sleep-wake schedule, avoiding stress when possible, eating a healthy diet, getting proper exercise, and following good sleep hygiene rules will usually help. Helpful dietary changes include a low-carbohydrate diet—especially avoiding any simple sugars—and reduced caffeine. Calcium supplements have been shown to reduce symptoms in some women.

Women with premenstrual symptoms may also have underlying circadian disturbances that cause them to waken too early in the morning or sleep too late. Bright light therapy, which involves sitting in front of a light box for an extended time in the morning or at night, has been reported to be effective in preventing some hormone-related sleep disorders. (Bright light therapy can also be useful for coping with wintertime depression, and for elderly people who don't get enough early morning activity to keep their biological clock attuned to the rhythms of the normal day. For more information, see page 258 in Chapter 14.)

Sleep restriction may reduce menses-related symptoms of depression, often in conjunction with antidepressants and psychiatric treatment when necessary. Sleep restriction therapy works in some cases of insomnia and depression and is discussed in Chapter 10.

(For more information on women and sleep, log on to www.sleepfoundation.org/publications/women.cfm.)

Pregnancy

My wife and I have four children, but she *had* them, and I had to stand aside as helpless as any other father and "coach." Much as we men may feel as though at times our partners are doing their best to make sure we feel their pain and all the other things that go with pregnancy, we get off lightly.

When I think of all the physical symptoms that pregnant women experience—morning sickness, cramps, varicose veins, and fetal movement—and the emotional changes—depression, anxiety, and worry—it's a wonder they can sleep at all. A National Sleep Foundation survey showed that 78 percent of women report more sleep disturbance during pregnancy than at any other time.

I'd like to think that there is some reassuring evolutionary reason for all of this sleeplessness—that the body is preparing women for the vigilance that characterizes a protective mother, or that it is disrupting her sleep so that she is prepared for nighttime feeding. But evolution hasn't caught up with the way we live now; this kind of routine discomfort is rarely tolerated in other aspects of life.

PREGNANCY AND THE NIGHT SHIFT

As you read in Chapter 4, the body does different things at different times of the day, and as you will read in Chapter 15, these normal physical processes often clash with the work schedules at our jobs. However, certain problems are unique to women.

A Danish study published in the July 2001 *American Journal of Obstetrics and Gynecology* shows that working the night shift increases by 35 percent the risk of delivering a child past its due date. For women at risk of having babies with low birth weight, working the night shift raises that risk to almost 80 percent.

The research team headed by Jin Liang Zhu, of Denmark's University of Aarhus, compared women who worked days only with women who worked only nights, and with those whose shifts rotated.

Women with fixed nighttime hours had the highest risk of delivering after their due dates, approximately one in six.

According to the researchers, "Night work may prolong the duration of pregnancy and reduce fetal growth, especially among industrial workers. Industrial workers with fixed night work had a high risk of post-term birth."

SLEEP BY TRIMESTER

An old folk adage describes the three trimesters as "weary, cheery, and dreary." This is borne out by the sleep profiles for each.

Weary.—the first three months: There is a greater tendency to sleep during this time than later in pregnancy or in the nonpregnant state. High levels of progesterone contribute to heightened feelings of sleepiness. There is more frequent urination, including at night. Sleep interruption causes daytime sleepiness. About 25 percent of women in the first trimester experience sleep disturbance.

Cheery.—the middle three months: Sleep is better than in the first trimester. Progesterone levels continue to rise but at a slower rate. The growing fetus exerts less pressure on the bladder, so urination decreases.

Dreary.—the home stretch: This is peak sleep-disturbance season. Physical discomfort increases from such complaints as heartburn, leg cramps, congested sinuses, and renewed pressure on the bladder, resulting in more bathroom visits. More women than men develop restless legs syndrome, generally, and 15 percent of women develop restless legs syndrome during the third trimester. It is very likely that this is a by-product of hormonal fluctuation, which can affect the work of the neuropathways in various ways that haven't been fully studied. Unfortunately, any medications used to treat this condition may be harmful to the fetus. However, the symptoms disappear in most of these new RLSers. Sleep is altered in 75 percent of women in the last trimester.

SOUNDS OF SWELLING

Well, not really. You can't hear bodily tissues engorging with fluids. All you can hear is the sound that they make when air passes through the ones in your airway when they are swollen, in the form of snoring.

Women who have never snored before often start in pregnancy because hormonal changes cause the nasal passages to swell, producing nonallergic rhinitis and blocking the airways as described in Chapter 5. The fact that this is first-time snoring and may be temporary doesn't mean it should be neglected. In the event of apnea, the oxygen supply to both mother and fetus is disrupted. Both are subject to the hormonal jolts of last-gasp resuscitation. And the spasms of sleep apnea can lead to excessive daytime sleepiness for mom.

Moreover, first-time snoring can cause changes in the airway tissues that will make mom more inclined to chronic snoring or apnea later on.

With all the warnings about smoking and pregnancy over the past couple of decades, it should surprise no one that other forms of compromised breathing also put the fetus at risk.

Snoring and sleep-disordered breathing have been linked to a twofold increase in preeclampsia in pregnancy. In addition, there are higher rates of hypertension and fetal growth reduction compared with nonsnorers. This has led some doctors and health care providers to carefully screen for snoring and sleep apnea in patients who are at high risk for preeclampsia especially when they suffer from conditions such as hypertension, obesity, or previous history of preeclampsia. The screening test may include urine and blood tests as well as a sleep study.

Sleep Tips during Pregnancy

1. Pamper yourself.
   - Take a warm shower or bath just before bed.
   - Ask your partner to massage your back, shoulders, and neck to help you relax.
2. Help blood flow to vital organs.
   - During the second and third trimester, sleep on your left side to allow better blood flow to the uterus, the kidneys, and the fetus.
   - Don't lie on your back except briefly.
3. Drink lots of fluids except before bedtime, but stay away from caffeine.
4. If you are prone to heartburn:
   - Stay away from excessive amounts of spicy foods, fried foods, and acidic foods.
   - Sleep with your upper body raised six to eight inches.
   - Avoid lying down for two hours after you eat.
5. Exercise.
6. If you are prone to nausea, eat small snacks of bland food and keep your stomach full.
7. Take naps.
8. If you experience a creeping or crawling feeling in your legs when you lie down—characteristic of restless legs syndrome—try to stretch, walk, or massage your legs, and be sure to tell your doctor.

AFTER THE BABY IS BORN

It is a measure of just how like other mammals people are that the sound of a baby crying is enough to make a nursing mother start to lactate. Nursing has come back into popular favor in recent years, and with good reason. That doesn't mean, however, that mom has to get up every time the baby needs to eat during the night. Breast pumps allow dad and the rest of the family to share some of the feeding chores as well as changing. There is a good possibility that postpartum depression is partially related to sleep deprivation, although I have no specific data. Depression can be serious, however, and at the first signs of the blues talk to your partner, family, friends, and doctor. I hope that you would *also alert your family and friends* to look for signs of depression. Suffice it to say that enlisting them to join in on postpartum chores to help mom sleep well is good for all parties, child included.

Change of Life, Change of Sleep

The observed changes in sleep associated with menopause can be broken down into the following categories: hot flashes, affective disorders, insomnia, and sleep-disordered breathing. I will address these individually.

HOT FLASHES

Given the fluctuations of mood, behavior, and sleep experience that come from the hormonal roller coaster of menstruation, it is only logical that the decline of those hormonal cycles should result in some swings of their own. In fact, lower levels of estrogen affect the hypothalamus, which as you know from earlier chapters plays a principal role in regulating your sleep cycles. The lower estrogen levels in effect send a false alarm to the brain that your body is too hot. Your body reacts as it would to a high fever. Neurotransmitters surge, including those insomnia-related culprits norepinephrine and serotonin, your heart pumps faster, blood vessels in your skin dilate so you can radiate heat, and you perspire.

This heat-releasing mechanism is a lifesaver—it keeps your body temperature down in the summer and when you exercise, but when there is a false alarm, it results in hot flashes. Your skin temperature can rise as much as 6 degrees centigrade or 11 degrees Fahrenheit. Men, think of how you would feel if your skin temperature shot up like that. Where's the fire?

Seventy to 80 percent of perimenopausal women have hot flashes, which last for about three minutes and go on for about one year although some women have them for several years.

Hormone replacement therapy has long been used to help ease the transition to menopause. It has been shown to increase REM sleep and deep sleep in the first one-third of sleep and also to improve sleep efficiency and decrease awakenings. Unfortunately, replacement therapy, has now been implicated as a risk factor for a number of serious conditions, including breast cancer, heart disease, and stroke. Newer types of pure progesterone, an estrogen patch, or alternative medications such as neurontin and serotonin reuptake inhibitors (SSRIs) may prove to be safer and more effective.

Depression and anxiety that coincide with menopause are thought to be related to many factors, not just hormonal change, but changing life circumstances, such as "empty-nest syndrome," including family issues such as marital change and career changes such as retirement.

Further complicating the picture are the connections between insomnia and chronic sleep deprivation with depression. Some studies have shown benefits from combining psychotherapy and medication. To these I would add sound sleep medicine principles, especially sleep hygiene. Each case should be treated individually.

MENOPAUSE AND INSOMNIA

Stressors are key to the development of both acute and chronic insomnia. As discussed in Chapter 10, a model of predisposition, precipitating factors, and perpetuating factors helps us understand how insomnia evolves. Within this model, menopause represents a "trifecta"—it can be all three Ps rolled into one. It's hard to know where one ends and the others begin. Suffice it to say that interruption or cessation of repetitive stressors that have affected your life for several days every month for 40 years can easily affect sleep behavior.

Regardless of whether you have the attitude that "this too shall pass," chronic insomnia from any cause should be evaluated and treated, as discussed in Chapter 10, starting with a thorough examination and sleep evaluation and history. Medical conditions and additional sleep disorders may exist that contribute to or totally explain the sleep complaint. If this is truly an insomnia related to menopause, a combination of behavioral and cognitive therapy and possibly medication may be recommended.

MENOPAUSE AND SLEEP-DISORDERED BREATHING

Every Breath You Take

Harriet, age 58, sat in front of me on her first visit and outlined her self-diagnosis and treatment plan—all in the first ten minutes of the interview. I listened and took a careful history and confirmed every detail of her self-diagnosis. Three years ago her husband had been diagnosed with sleep apnea. At the time, Harriet made it her business to learn everything about the disorder. Now postmenopausal, she recognized the signs and symptoms: snoring, weight gain, and excessive daytime sleepiness.

Two months after I confirmed and treated her obstructive apnea, she returned with her husband to report success of treatment and to make a request: They wondered if I could arrange for a special CPAP "Y" connector that would push in air from one machine to synchronize their breathing during sleep. Talk about togetherness! I told them I would put it on my list of interesting research concepts.

This was not an isolated case. Several times a year I see a post-menopausal woman who recognizes her own sleep apnea as a result of a treated partner. Perhaps all postmenopausal women should view an educational video on sleep apnea during their routine doctor visit.

Snoring, sometimes severe, is a common complaint among peri-menopausal women. It may be caused by changes in body fat distribution or behavior that alter the shape of the upper airway. The known hormone changes of menopause may actually have enough impact on the upper airway to suggest formulating a different set of risk factors for apnea in women compared with that for men. Severe snoring may also carry separate risks for medical illness as discussed in Chapter 5.

Sleep apnea occurs in one in four women over the age of 65. The increase in abdominal girth during menopause may explain the three to four times increase in sleep apnea in menopausal women. A decrease in progesterone is also suspected as a cause for the increased incidence. Untreated apnea is now well known to be associated with hypertension, stroke, and heart disease.

Treatment of Menopause-Related Breathing Disorders

Menopause-related sleep disturbances can be diminished by following general sleep hygiene rules, with particular attention to controlling your bedroom temperature, adjusting the light, and using comfortable (preferably cotton) bed linen. Eliminating caffeine, sugar, and alcohol from your diet should also be considered. As mentioned in Chapter 7, treatments such as weight-loss, CPAP therapy, and/or an oral appliance can be used to deal with altered airways. An evaluation by an ENT (ear, nose, and throat) specialist is advised. As with many sleep disorders, the combination of antidepressants, supportive psychotherapy and behavioral therapy should be considered.

Special Considerations in Pregnancy and Menopause
RESTLESS LEGS SYNDROME (RLS) AND
PERIODIC LIMB MOVEMENT DISORDER (PLMD)

According to a National Sleep Foundation 2002 poll, 18 percent of women reported symptoms of RLS a few nights a week or more. As previously mentioned, about 15 percent of women who are not normally prone to RLS experience it in the third trimester. Because of the associated insomnia and disrupted sleep, RLS can lead to daytime sleepiness with all the associated physical and psychosocial consequences. In addition to depression and anxiety, one study showed that 42 percent of those affected with RLS reported that it interfered with their personal relationships.

Since RLS is associated with low iron and/or folate levels, women are particularly at risk for the condition. About 80 percent of women who have RLS have limb movements that disturb their sleep and cause daytime sleepiness (PLMD). Details of both conditions and treatment are discussed in Chapter 9. Most cases related to pregnancy resolve themselves after delivery. All treatments should be discussed with your doctor since some of the medications used for treatment may cause damage to the fetus or may damage the liver.

Medical Conditions

More women than men suffer from such painful ailments as migraine, tension headaches, chronic fatigue syndrome, and fibromyalgia by a margin of 58-42 percent, according to a 1996 National Sleep Foundation Gallup Poll, and these probably also interfere with their sleep. Women also suffer a higher incidence of arthritic pain and discomfort from gastric reflux than men. These conditions, too, can compromise quality sleep.

NIGHTTIME SLEEP-RELATED EATING DISORDER

This is an uncommon condition, but 66 percent of those who have it are women. Eating can occur during sleepwalking and there is usually no recall of the event. This behavior can be caused by awakenings related to another sleep disorder such as leg movement disorder or can be related to medication such as some antidepressants. We treat it as an insomnia, using medication and behavioral therapy.

General Recommendations for Treatment of Sleep Disorders in Women

- See a doctor if your sleep is disrupted or if you have excessive daytime sleepiness.
- Getting older is not an adequate explanation for sleeping problems and you should not take it for granted that you will sleep badly for the rest of your life. If you are troubled by daytime sleepiness, a sleep study may be required to rule out major sleep disorders.
- If you are aware that you snore and you get pregnant, mention it to your doctor. Blood pressure and urine evaluations are considered essential and you may need a sleep study if there are signs of sleep-disordered breathing.

As should be clear by now, the field of sleep medicine is developing very rapidly, and like other fields of rapidly growing knowledge, new ideas enter the mix all the time. This is particularly true with clinical medicine, which is both art and science as opposed to laboratory research. I mention this because of a paper I recently read by Dr. Daniel Kahneman of Princeton University, published in *Science* and reported in *The New York Times,* which looked at the lives of 909 working women in Texas and examined, among other things, what made them happy, sad, or stressed during a typical day.

Of great interest to me was the way the study was designed. Using a novel questionnaire called the Day Reconstruction Method, the women were instructed to keep a diary of an average of 14 activities that they performed for about one hour throughout the day, such as reading the paper, commuting, interacting with children, cooking, or caring for a family member. The next day they reviewed the diary and tried to relive the experience emotionally, assigning a number based on a scale to rate their enjoyment of each activity.

It was no surprise to me that sleep, or the lack of sleep as recorded in their diaries had a major impact on the results. Most women woke up a little grumpy. The lack of sleep was one of two major factors that affected their ratings of the activities and of their overall happiness. Activities rated high on the list for what makes women happy included intimate relationships, socializing, exercising, and watching TV. Women who slept poorly reported less enjoyment from activities on the whole.

It occurred to me that this method would enhance the standard sleep diary because it could help track how both mind and body are responding to life's daily stressors. The value of such a record was brought home to me when I reviewed the case of Leah, Rebecca, and Rebecca's daughters presented earlier in this chapter. All three generations of women were experiencing sleep disturbances for different reasons and occasionally at the same time. Their long-term and monthly hormone changes probably had a profound effect on sleep not only for the individual but also for the others in the family. As we heard from Leah, her sleep disturbance evolved over time and became chronic and dynamic in response to life stressors. This points to the importance of evaluating and treating any sleep disturbance that continues for more than one to two weeks.

Women's incidence of obstructive sleep apnea and leg movement disorders also probably needs to be studied in all age groups and not compared only with previous studies in the general population. We know that when it comes to sleep, men and women are not created equal and we need to evaluate the women's sleep disorders with this in mind.

14

OLDER, WISER, AND SLEEPIER

Ralph worked at our hospital as an oncologic pharmacist. When he was 66 years old, he was looking forward to his planned Florida retirement with something less than enthusiasm.

One of the things that bothered him was that he was fearful of driving to Florida because he was worried he might doze off at the wheel. I examined him and found he was overweight, that he snored, and that he had a very crowded airway. After the sleep study confirmed apnea, I put him on CPAP treatment, and in his words, "saved his retirement life." Each year when he visits his old Brooklyn home, he updates me on his condition.

Prior to Ralph's trip in 2002, his New York cardiologist reported a jump in his heart ejection fraction—that is, the pump strength of his heart muscle. Ralph can feel the improvement from the CPAP treatment. Exercise has become easier now that he is sleeping well, and he has lost enough weight to require a new wardrobe.

This improvement has yielded other benefits. In addition to his depression lifting, because of the improvement in the condition of his heart, he became a better candidate for surgery that had been postponed. He has two new titanium knees, allowing him to walk better; a repaired prostate, complete with easy urine flow; and he has reduced his daily intake of pills by 50 percent.

He was proud to report that on the drive up to New York from Florida he was able to last longer at the wheel and take fewer, more leisurely pit stops instead of more emergency stops. There was no need for naps every two hours as there had been in his pre-CPAP days. He even felt alert enough to drive alongside an 82-year-old neighbor whose boasts about his own health used to depress Ralph even more. He was most excited, however, about getting his sister on CPAP after she complained to him about classic symptoms. "She went straight to her doctor and told him, 'I know why I am sleepy—my brother told me.'" Ralph was right.

Are You a Baby Boomer Trying to Cope with Aging Parents?

You can play a part in making your parents' advancing years more comfortable. There are specific symptoms pertinent to sleep disorders that doctors should know when taking a medical history, but many elderly people will not relate them. You can take the first step toward treatment for your loved one by paying attention to the following:

1. What do they mostly complain about?
   Excessive sleepiness

   Inability to go to sleep when they want to

   Early-morning awakening

   Two or three of the above

2. Do they get enough sleep based on your knowledge of their needs?
3. Have their sleeping hours changed noticeably from what you think are their usual hours?
4. Do they complain about bedroom noise, too much light, or uncomfortable temperatures?
5. Do they have an underlying medical or psychiatric illness that you suspect might be contributing to the sleep disturbance?
6. Are they drinking an unaccustomed amount of caffeine or alcohol or are they taking prescription or nonprescription drugs?

7. Are they complaining of snoring or twitching, which may indicate the presence of primary sleep disorders such as sleep apnea, restless legs syndrome, or periodic limb movements?
8. Are they watching TV in bed, or falling asleep in front of the TV? Are they taking daytime naps?

Americans are living longer than ever, and as their lives get longer, their hours of sleep get shorter.

The number of Americans aged 65 and older climbed above 34.9 million in 2000, compared with 3.1 million in 1900. And it has been projected that the population aged 65 to 74 will have grown 74 percent between 1990 and 2020.

When the nation was founded, the average American could expect to live to the age of 35. Life expectancy at birth had increased to 47.3 by 1900 and in 2000 stood at 76.9.

In 1990, 1 out of every 6,667 people was 100 years or older. In 2000, the ratio was 1 out of every 5,578 people. The oldest old (persons 85 years old and over) are a small but rapidly growing group, comprising just over 1 percent of the American population in 1994. Overall, the oldest old are projected to be the fastest-growing part of the elderly population as we move further into the 21st century.

Baby Boomers and the National Sleep Deficit

The baby boom generation is about to start retiring. The Social Security trust fund may or may not run a deficit but for many of the boomers, their sleep certainly will. Given the problems elderly people have in sleeping, the national sleep deficit is going to skyrocket.

Elderly patients typically have trouble falling asleep and spend less time in the deeper stages of sleep, in addition to getting less sleep overall. They have irregular sleep-wake times and nap during the day, which may contribute to insomnia. National Institute on Aging research on over 9,000 persons aged 65 years and above recorded at least one chronic sleep complaint in half of both men and women.

Restless legs syndrome and periodic limb movement disorder, sleep apnea, excessive daytime sleepiness and the full range of associated complaints—are all more common among the elderly than among younger people. Sleep disorder evaluations and studies for older people must concentrate particularly hard on poor sleep habits because many of the elderly have a less formal routine to anchor their days than they had when they were younger.

In addition, aggravating factors may include acute and chronic medical illnesses, medication, psychiatric disorders, and changes in their circadian rhythms. Their difficulties may be further compounded by attempts to medicate themselves with alcohol and over-the-counter preparations. Well-intended, commonsense advice from health care workers, social workers, and family members may miss the mark for a very specific and individual sleep problem. Stubbornness about seeking help is as much a culprit as following bad advice—older people are prone to depression and denial about their changing circumstances and they don't like to acknowledge that their children in particular may know better than they do.

It is common knowledge that elderly bones are more fragile than younger ones, but so are all organ systems. The consequences of chronic sleep problems often add a veil of complexity to virtually all medical problems. The elderly are already at greater risk of serious injury from falls, and this risk is compounded by sleep deprivation or chronic use of sedating medications. Sleep-disordered breathing will take a more severe toll on the cardiovascular, pulmonary, and central nervous systems of the elderly. With so many elderly people already suffering from hypertension, they don't need sleep apnea, too. Severe sleep disruption often complicates the task of nursing home placement, especially if there is an added diagnosis of dementia.

Aging Time Clock

In Chapter 2, you learned about the suprachiasmatic nuclei, or SCN, small brain structures located near the pituitary gland at the base of the brain. These constitute, as noted, the brain's "biological clock" where the circadian rhythms are controlled. Signals from sunlight help set the timing of the SCN, which in turn affect many other physiological functions.

As you age, your brain's time clock keeps working. However, the pathways for signals to and from the clock change, which alters your response to circadian rhythms. While your digestion and other bodily functions change, one of the most obvious of those changes will be in how you sleep—your urge to nap, your sensitivity to noise and other stimuli, an earlier time of awakening.

As the chart below indicates, sleep changes as we age in terms of both the amount of each stage of sleep and the timing of that sleep throughout the night.

Sleep Through the Ages

Type of Sleep	% Sleep for Infant	% Sleep for Young Child	% Sleep for Young Adult	% Sleep for Elderly Adult
Stage 1	<5%	<5%	<5%	8–15%
Stage 2	25–30%	40–45%	45–55%	70–80%
Delta Sleep	20%	25–30%	13–23%	0–5%
REM Sleep	50%	25–30%	20–25%	20%

Compared with young adults, the elderly tend to have, more stage-1 sleep reflecting more awakenings, less deep sleep, and more stage-2 sleep.

There are other important differences in sleep in the elderly compared with young children and adults as discussed below.

SLEEP STAGES OF CHILDREN

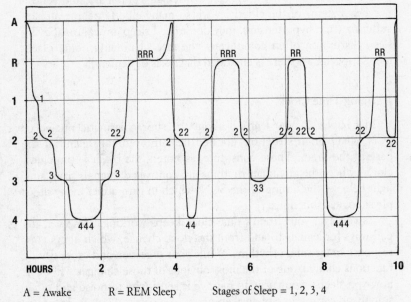

A = Awake   R = REM Sleep   Stages of Sleep = 1, 2, 3, 4

The panel above shows episodes of uninterrupted and deep sleep in the young child. You can see the increased amount of deep stage-3 and -4 sleep and the larger amount of REM sleep over the entire night. Most of the deep sleep occurs early in the night.

SLEEP STAGES OF ADULTS

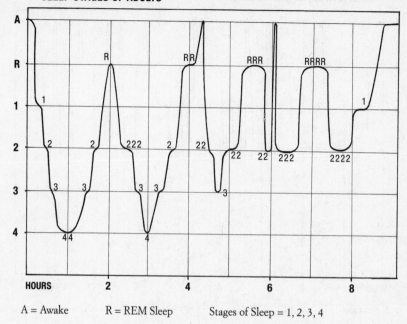

A = Awake   R = REM Sleep   Stages of Sleep = 1, 2, 3, 4

This panel shows how adults start to lose deep sleep, have reduced REM sleep, and have more frequent awakenings than children. On arriving home after a late-night drive if you tried to carry a sleeping adult out of the backseat of the car you would find that they would probably wake up, and possibly object, in contrast to the lead-weighted slumber of the tiny tot.

SLEEP STAGES OF THE ELDERLY

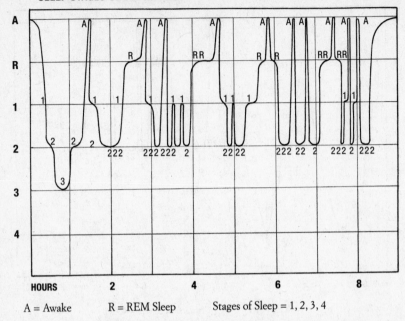

A = Awake   R = REM Sleep   Stages of Sleep = 1, 2, 3, 4

The most striking change is seen in the elderly sleep pattern with frequent awakenings all through the night and especially toward the morning hours. Also there is very little deep sleep. The total sleep time is also reduced reflecting the poor quality of sleep not the need for less.

Getting On and Getting a Good Night's Sleep

While elderly persons tend to get less sleep at night than younger people, we can't assume that they need less of it. They wake up at night more frequently and suffer from increased daytime sleepiness as a result, which they make up for by taking naps.

The elderly generally still get their REM sleep. However, deep non-REM sleep is often drastically reduced or nonexistent. This is the phase of sleep that is associated with the secretion of human growth hormone (HGH). Whether growth hormone levels are reduced because of diminished deep non-REM sleep or deep non-REM sleep is reduced because of secretion of the hormone is lower is unknown. There's a chicken-or-egg problem here. However, there is no question that many people associate the lower levels of HGH with advancing age, and many people are trying to reverse the aging process with injections of the hormone. We do not know, however, what long-term effects these shots will have on the body. They may go beyond the desired tissue restoration to the unwanted growth of tissues in organs such as the heart, which can present a long-run danger.

With some significant exceptions, elderly persons tend to go to bed earlier and as a result wake up earlier than they did before. There would be nothing wrong with this if they started getting up at 6 A.M., where they formerly woke up at 7 A.M., read the paper, and led a productive day. The problem is that they often awaken spontaneously at 4:30 A.M. when the world is dark and lonely. If they don't go to sleep much earlier to compensate for this early awakening, they become sleep deprived. Daytime napping may make the problem worse by delaying sleep onset at bedtime.

Delayed sleep phase syndrome, which was described in Chapter 2 in conjunction with our coin collector, is another problem for elderly people. It occurs when the waking day shifts later into the night and the sleeping night extends later and later into the daylight hours. This may stem from a natural propensity toward a night owl schedule that in younger days was held in check by greater responsiveness to daylight and the responsibilities of work or raising children. Without this kind of routine, the possibility of a social life becomes more and more remote, as the following indicates.

Same Home Different Time Zones—Advanced Sleep Phase Syndrome and the Elderly Couple

The sleep problems of elderly parents can be a source of stress for their middle-aged children. A friend of mine despairs regularly over the state of his parents' life together in their "golden years."

"My mother was always a night owl," he says. "Raising four children, however, didn't give her much time to indulge herself. She waited till after everyone went to bed and stayed up reading the paper she didn't have time for." This "eagle" behavior—stretching one's inborn night owl behavior to encompass the demands of raising a young family of larks—is described in detail in Chapter 4.

In later years, as my friend describes it, after the children grew up, as the broadcast hours of television extended later and channels grew more numerous, television played a greater part in her solitary evenings. She frequently fell asleep on the couch and it would be hours before she finally dragged herself off to bed.

"My father was always more of a morning person, and still is," my friend continues. While he still works at home, in his early 80s his productivity is way down. The trouble is, however, that because my mother sleeps late every morning, they aren't very good companions for each other. Their decreasing mobility forces them to rely more and more on one another, but their mismatched schedules and the decrease in stimulation lead to inertia on split shifts."

He went on to describe his feelings of sadness and helplessness when his numerous attempts to help put them back in synch with one another and with the larger world were frustrated by what appeared to be fixed behavior.

The first step to the treatment was to help Mom, Dad, and my friend understand the problem. Dad's behavior, for example, could be compared to that of an early-morning-shift worker. Shift workers experience a similar kind of isolation when they miss the company of their spouse, children, partners, or family. Mom on the other hand could be thought of as living in another time zone. The out-of-synch schedules had become quite fixed over time and obviously added stress to the golden years.

I explained that we usually define a sleep disorder in terms of the negative effects it has on the individual's life, although this certainly could be extended to a couple's relationship, or even to family sleep disorder. The fix would require considerable effort and compromise on both sides. One or both would have to shift their sleep phase.

Dad could shift his advanced sleep phase by working in the vicinity of artificial bright light at night and going to bed and getting up an hour or two later every day (see the end of the chapter for a description of bright light therapy). Morning appointments or a planned walk or breakfast with Dad, might give Mom more reason to get up. Exposure to early-morning bright sunlight would help reset her delayed sleep phase by starting the day earlier and going to bed earlier. Greater structure in their lives in the form of more shared tasks and responsibilities could probably help create more positive interaction, making their sleep-wake schedule and last years together more satisfactory.

My middle-aged friend sums it up this way: "I still haven't finished raising my children, and I haven't finished raising myself. I wish I could do more for my parents. I also wish they would do more for themselves. I just hope I will do better at their age than they have done for themselves."

Unfortunately, my friends' parents didn't recognize the slow change in sleep patterns and drifted further apart, Dad shift working and Mom in a different time zone. By understanding how this evolved he can help them and himself and do more than just wish and hope.

Just Like Younger People, Only Worse

The factors that disrupt the sleep of younger people—noise, light, diet, and many others—are also factors in the sleeping-waking lives of the elderly, but to an even greater extent.

Poor Sleep Habits

As should be clear by now, sleep in the elderly suffers from a combination of wear and tear on the software, as a result of poor sleeping habits, and on the hardware, as a result of advancing age. Organs, bones, skin, and other tissues lose their resiliency as we get older. Without the regulation of responsibilities, a daytime schedule and routine, something similar happens to sleep. The 24-hour day loses its underlying support structure and shape. As we saw in the case of the aging couple recounted above, the discipline of job and family does for the sleep-wake cycles what exercise does for muscles. When it stops, the tendency toward regular sleep and wakefulness loses its tone. Routine starts to fray.

At this point, efforts to compensate for change may initiate a vicious cycle of new behavior, which aggravates the problem. Without thinking, we might compensate for afternoon sleepiness by drinking a cup of coffee, which never used to be part of our routine. As the coffee's effects last into the evening, we may take a drink of alcohol to calm down. But this self-medication doesn't deal with the underlying problem; in fact, it makes it worse. Alcohol, while initially sedating, inhibits deep sleep and promotes arousal as the night wears on. Excessive wakeful time in bed may cause excessive daytime sleepiness, microsleeps, and more naps.

Illness

Arthritis, prostate problems, and heart, gastrointestinal, and pulmonary diseases—the whole menu of geriatric indignities—disrupt sleep. Pain and discomfort make it harder to get to sleep and shorten its duration. Neurodegenerative disorders, particularly Alzheimer's disease and Parkinson's disease, are also very disruptive to the sleep cycle.

Medications
WHEN PILLS COLLIDE

A 70-year-old man started his consultation with me by dumping a plastic shopping bag full of medication on the table. He then declared, "My doctor wants you to fix my sleeping problem."

One by one he went through the meds. He held a bottle of Benadryl in an arthritic hand. "This one is for a rash on my legs," he said. Then he picked up a second bottle. "A few days after I started taking it my urine slowed down, and he figured out that it was my prostate reacting to the first one."

He put down the two bottles and grabbed a third. "Unfortunately, the drug I got from my arthritis specialist interacted with the pill used to calm down the prostate inflammation, so I had to start *this* one," referring to a prescription nonsteroidal anti-inflammatory. "Since he was afraid my stomach would bleed from that one, he put me on an antacid. But that gave me a rash, so I ended up right where I started!

"To make matters worse, I started urinating more at night, and all that waking up all night makes me sleepy during the day."

I asked him, "When do you take your pills?" He said that he had a schedule for taking them from 10 A.M. through 10 P.M., his bedtime. I had him line up the pills in the quantities and order in which he took them. He lined up 10 pills. "Show me what you do," I said.

In re-creating his medication routine, we counted four extra glasses of water that he drank with his pills between 10 A.M. and 10 P.M., on top of whatever he drinks with dinner and throughout the evening.

The fix was easy. Since the rash was already fading, we reduced the number of pills and rescheduled them so that he did not have to take pills or drink fluids after 7 P.M. The rash disappeared and he slept better than he had before the rash started.

Of course, water is not the only sleep-disrupting factor associated with pill taking. That medicine cabinet is full of powerful chemicals with individual side effects and properties that may clash with one another. Some antidepressants (particularly the commonly prescribed drugs called SSRIs, or selective serotonin reuptake inhibitors), decongestants, bronchodilators, antihypertensives, and corticosteroids are stimulants that can make it difficult to begin or remain sleeping. Nighttime use of diuretics—medications that make you urinate more—entails repeated trips to the bathroom. However, the quality of sleep when taking medications is not your sole concern. The quality of waking life is just as important. Medications and other substances that can either interfere with your sleep or change your level of alertness when awake include the following:

Drugs and foods that may interfere with sleep

- Some antidepressants, such as Prozac, which may alter appetite and make sleep more difficult
- Decongestants containing pseudoephedrine
- Cold medications containing decongestants
- Foods containing caffeine such as chocolate
- Dieuretics
- Nicotine

Drugs and foods that may induce sleepiness

- Antihistamines
- Beta-blockers
- Certain cold medications that may contain sedating components (read the labels carefully to look for warnings)
- Certain antidepressants
- Tranquilizers
- Alcohol (should not be used to get to sleep)
- Some herbal remedies
- L-dopa

Psychiatric Problems

We all know an older person (or at very least know someone related to an older person) who is affected by a psychiatric or degenerative neurological disease such as Alzheimer's. There is a ripple effect. The day is usually disrupted by the disease or by the medication used to treat it and this daytime disruption all too often carries over into the night.

In Chapter 10 we reviewed the role of mind, body, and the central nervous system in the cause of insomnia and this model applies even more so to the elderly. Anxiety, psychosis, and dementia all have complications associated with sleep disruption. Insomnia is common in the elderly and in elderly patients with major depression very common (it is found in 30 to 70 percent of this population). Diminished physical abilities, isolation, deaths of loved ones, and giving up the family home are all causes of depression and sleeping problems. Nighttime arousals and early-morning awakening may be severely exacerbated among the elderly when they are depressed. As in every other sleep disorder when it comes to psychiatric sleep disorders among the elderly, day predicts the night and night predicts the day. Evaluating and treating the entire 24-hour behavior gives the best results.

Primary Sleep Disorders and the Elderly

Any disruption of sleep will have a more profound effect on the patient or the individual organ systems when the parts are affected by disease or age. Things like joint pain and prostate problems begin to add up. Add joint pain to a sleep disorder and the disruption is compounded. The person's daytime behavior will, of course, reflect the disturbed sleep.

Primary sleep disorders are associated with aging. They cause all types of unwanted behaviors, from wandering to falling out of bed and disrupting the sleep of all those within earshot. I see this all the time during my rounds in the hospital and the staff easily recognizes the pattern: sleep all day, up all night.

Sleep apnea and other disordered breathing during sleep in the elderly deserve special mention. In previous chapters we have dealt with sleep apnea, restless legs syndrome, and various parasomnias. While these conditions are found among most age groups, they are more prevalent in older people and the special considerations of the elderly warrant further comment.

SLEEP-DISORDERED BREATHING AND THE ELDERLY

Obviously, a great number of our elderly populations are prone to a variety of serious medical problems that may result in sleep-disordered breathing. However, as patients and their physicians concentrate on the treatment of the primary disease, they may overlook the presence of the incidental condition, which may exacerbate their problems in the long run.

Risk factors for sleep-disordered breathing in the elderly include hypothyroidism, neurodegenerative disorders—especially Parkinson's disease, stroke, cardiovascular disorders, or any lung disease. Mechanical disorders of the lung and chest wall, such as severe emphysema, make breathing more difficult both during the day and at night.

Treatment of sleep apnea in the elderly is basically the same as in others. If a heart or lung disease patient also has apnea, CPAP therapy will likely be enriched with the addition of oxygen. The need for supplemental oxygen will be determined during a sleep study by measuring blood oxygen levels. In the event that CPAP is indicated for a patient with dementia, it may take some time and patience to help the person tolerate the mask since he or she may be confused or stubborn. Successful treatment in this group is possible since other special needs groups such as children with Down syndrome have been shown to tolerate CPAP therapy.

RESTLESS LEGS SYNDROME AND PERIODIC LIMB MOVEMENT DISORDER

As described in Chapter 9, restless legs syndrome is characterized by intense aching and possibly by a "creepy-crawly" sensation when the person is at rest. The person feels a strong urge to keep moving the legs or to get up and walk around to relieve the discomfort.

Restless legs syndrome may significantly interfere with sleep. One of the most severe cases in my practice was seen in a patient with neurological disease. A 78-year-old man with early dementia started to pace up and down the hall around bedtime. He lived in a duplex with his wife, his daughter, her husband, and their two-year-old. The episodes were very dramatic, with loud voices and heavy-footed marching that disturbed all on the first floor.

What followed was an emotional and difficult discussion with the family regarding the possibility of worsening dementia and nursing home placement.

Fortunately, a more focused sleep history and evaluation proved helpful. Taking the history is difficult in someone with dementia; it's almost always the family members or attendants who provide the key information. In this case the daughter remarked that her father would reach down intermittently and rub his legs during the pacing marathons.

This is a key feature of restless legs syndrome. Going on that presumptive diagnosis and with the help of a very thorough workup at the hospital, I started treatment with Mirapex, a dopamine agonist. The results were dramatic. His pacing stopped, his sleep improved and even the two-year-old slept better as a result of the return to a peaceful routine.

Periodic limb movement disorder, another primary sleep disorder among the elderly, may accompany presleep or daytime restless legs syndrome or occur only during sleep. The leg movements or arm movements result in disruption of continuous sleep, often occurring hundreds of times throughout the night. They typically produce many brief arousals that disrupt sleep organization and decrease the amount of time in the deeper stages of sleep. This arousal from sleep may be very tightly linked to the movements and when it occurs often enough causes sleep disruption analogous to someone poking the sleeper on the shoulder every 40 seconds, saying, "Hey get up." You can see the disruption of peaceful sleep by reviewing the impact of leg movements on the sleeping brain on page 161 in Chapter 9 on leg movement disorder.

The delay in getting to sleep, and sleep disruption from periodic limb movements during sleep, will cause daytime sleepiness. Risk factors for these two disorders include increasing age, neurological disease, hematological disease, kidney failure, and iron deficiency. Up to 30 percent of elderly persons have measurable periodic leg movements during sleep. Not every case requires treatment; the total number of events and the impact of the movements on good sleep determine treatment.

In addition to treating the underlying disease, the limb movements and discomfort can be treated with warm soaks of the affected limb, exercise, or additional medication. It is important to remember the elderly may have a sluggish metabolism adding an additional risk for medication side effects.

Carbidopa-levodopa (Simemet), Pramipexole (Mirapex), Pergolide (Permax), or a bedtime dose of a benzodiazepine, Clorazepam, or a low-potency opiate, such as codeine or oxycodone (Roxicodone), may also help. Bromocriptine (Parlodel), carbamazepine (Tegretol), and clonazepam (Klonopin) are other options. Clonazepam, however, deserves special mention since it may contribute to falls and injury if the unmonitored elderly person awakens at night and attempts to get out of bed. To minimize the possibility of confused arousals and falls, follow the general guidelines and sleep hygiene rules as discussed below. If the daytime behavior is erratic and medication is required for restless legs or related insomnia, consider either direct bedside observation or a monitoring device similar to that used for infants and children. Specific treatment with medication and potential side effects are discussed in Chapter 9.

Information and support are available from organizations such as the Restless Legs Syndrome Foundation (Web site: http://www.rls.org).

The Heart-Lung Pump

To appreciate the special dangers of sleep-disordered breathing for the elderly or anyone with heart or lung disease, it helps to envision the mechanical functioning of the heart and lungs.

Briefly, the heart pumps blood to all tissues and organs, one of which is the lungs. A bellows-type pump, consisting of the ribs and muscles that comprise the chest wall, also drives the lungs. We all experience a change in blood pressure, oxygen level, and heart rate in some stages of sleep. That is quite normal and when all systems are operating normally we awaken refreshed unaware of the adjustments and normal compensations.

However, the heart or lung pump can be damaged directly, for example, by a heart attack or the hereditary type of emphysema. Damage can also occur indirectly as a result of blocking the outflow from the pump as in heart strain from hypertension or lung disease from cigarette smoking. Like any pump, blocking outflow will cause the pump to strain and eventually fail. When this happens to the heart "pump," it is called congestive heart failure (CHF) and when it happens to the lungs it is called chronic obstructive pulmonary disease (COPD). Both diseases are more common in the elderly. According to the National Heart, Lung and Blood Institute (NHLBI), 4.8 million Americans have CHF, with the highest rate of 10 percent found in those in the 70-and-older group. There are an estimated 14 million patients in the United States with COPD and worldwide it is the fourth leading cause of death for this age group.

For people with any of these conditions, sleep-disordered breathing can make sleep downright hazardous.

During the day, patients with borderline heart or lung function stay out of severe trouble because they have some higher-brain control over pump function. They can slow down if they are walking too fast, reducing demands on the heart and lungs for oxygen. They can sit and put their feet up, or urinate at the first urge and thereby limit fluid overload. They can sit up instead of lying down, so that gravity can help the chest wall and lung pump. In many cases these compensations during the day in addition to a long list of medications, keeps them functioning and just out of the danger zone.

However, the sleeping brain offers far less protection. When the vigilant waking brain is turned off and unable to send recovery signals, the patient begins to react in other ways. Unlike the healthy heart or lung pump, the damaged systems also contribute to abnormal compensations. This may result in more severe sleep apnea, restless sleep with insomnia, or a worsening of their underlying disease. The critical difference, compared with those with no heart or lung disease, is an absent or blunted response to the changes in their heart rate, oxygen levels, and blood pressure as they fluctuate marginally out of the danger zone.

Patients or their family members describe a number of symptoms that are warning signs of failing systems. They cite shortness of breath when walking, swelling legs, and a seeming inability to lie down flat because breathing becomes difficult.

As the heart or lung condition gets worse, patients with more severe problems will start to experience, for example, slow progressive weight gain, leg swelling, lethargy, and shortness of breath during the day. The body loses the capacity for physical activity. Eventually, patients may experience severe cardiopulmonary insufficiency or heart-lung failure. This is a 24-hour failure, however, and the night portion is often not fully recognized or experienced by the patient.

On my morning rounds it is not uncommon for me to see an elderly patient attached to a ventilator who was admitted to the ICU the night before for respiratory failure. The family generally thinks he or she has had a heart attack or some other catastrophic event. Listening to family members, I will hear a familiar tale unfold: progressive shortness of breath during the day, leg swelling, and severe snoring. However, it usually takes an emergency to get these patients to see a doctor. And by then it is "too late."

What we are seeing is not always a heart attack or any other sudden organ failure but, rather, an indication that the slow deterioration in the two major pump systems has progressed to the point where they are overloaded. In fact, the relative stress to the system is not in itself exceptional, but only comparable to what the patients would experience from walking too fast. However, because the patients are asleep and don't realize it, they can't adjust by stopping to rest or putting their feet up, as they would if they were awake. For many weeks or months, the body has compensated by prompting a brief arousal from sleep for a brief episode, during which the output of the cardiopulmonary system rises to levels high enough to temporarily stave off failure. Eventually, however, the low oxygen states night after night catch up with them, and that's when they end up in the ICU. Fortunately this overload is often reversible to a great extent with diuretics, oxygen, or water pills, or medication to help the heart pump. Patients are usually off the respirator in a couple of days.

REM-Behavior Disorder

REM-behavior disorder occurs most commonly in elderly persons. Unfortunately it is often misunderstood and assumed to be a behavioral problem. REM-behavior disorder is discussed in greater detail in Chapter 11. Underlying this disorder is a faulty "REM switch," which allows muscle activity during dreaming that ordinarily wouldn't happen. Patients may thrash about in bed, strike out at bed partners, and occasionally injure themselves or others. Treatment in the elderly may prove difficult since the main treatments include a bedtime dose of a long-acting benzodiazepine such as clonazepam. These drugs may have significant side effects such as dizziness and confusion. This is not the best choice, for example, for a fragile, light-sleeping, snoring, agitated elderly person with lung disease. Treatments must be individualized after a very careful inventory of the patients' medications, underlying medical conditions, and psychiatric history. Also a sleep study may be necessary to rule out the existence of other sleep disorders.

General Treatment Considerations

The combination of presenting problems and underlying disease states in the elderly present a real challenge. As with any sleep disorder, good sleep hygiene applies. Two recurrent themes throughout this book are:

- A healthy existence is a 24-hour-a-day, 7-day-a-week concern.
- Along with diet and exercise, good sleep hygiene is one of the keys to a healthy state.

When younger people ignore these three elements it is like burning the money they need to live on, but they have enough that they feel they can afford it. However, in older people, their physical resources, like their financial ones are often more limited.

Golden Sleep Rules for Golden Agers

Note to Caregivers: If patients cannot do these things for themselves, try to follow these rules on their behalf.

1. *Keep a regular, moderate schedule.* Sleep, diet, and exercise need some planning and common sense. Don't jog in the rain, don't eat sirloin steaks before bed, and don't sleep whenever you want to.

2. *Stay active.* Don't sit around all day. This will help you keep your weight steady and get you good and tired right in time for sleep.

3. *Get out in the sun, weather permitting, as early as you can,* although you should protect your eyes and skin as usual. If it is overcast outside, or the weather is unpleasant, at least open the curtains and keep them open. Don't forget that the timing of daylight is one of the keys to setting your biological clock. During the short days of winter, or in the event of a sleep phase problem, in which you rise later in the day than most people, a sleep specialist can help with the design and timing of an artificial lighting scheme.

   Bright light therapy has proven to be beneficial for several types of sleep disorders. If you have advanced sleep phase syndrome (ASPS), you may notice that you wake up too early every morning and feel sleepy way before your desired bedtime. Conversely, delayed sleep phase syndrome (DSPS) is when you have difficulty getting to sleep and then sleep late into the morning. The insomnia noted in sleep phase disorders is associated with the attempt to or urge to sleep at the wrong time relative to your internal clock or the circadian drive to sleep. Getting up early, and getting a strong light signal, as for example in a brightly lit climate, is one method to maintain healthy circadian timing although the elderly often have difficulty getting out and about.

   Selective application of bright light therapy in the morning (to correct a late sleep phase delay) or in the evening (to correct an early sleep phase advance) has been very effective in "resetting" patients' internal clock to coincide with a more reasonable sleep routine. The artificial light reaches the retina and eventually helps reset the SCN. There are many light boxes on the market, which can simulate bright light of day and help start the bodies' time clock ticking on a more desirable schedule. The treatment is used every day and at the same time, for between one-quarter and three-quarters of an hour. The user does not have to stare at the light, but can watch TV, read, or do chores in the vicinity of the light. The light intensity is about 2,500 lux, which is about five times as bright as a well-lit room. However, if you are on medication, have light-sensitive skin, or have problems with your eyes, talk to your doctor before you use light therapy.

4. *Make the bedroom sleep-friendly.* Do this according to your personal tastes and preferences. What makes you feel at peace and relaxed? Surround yourself with things that give you comfort. Don't forget, however, that this is supposed to be a nice place to sleep, not a place to do daytime activities. If you live in one room, set it up so that there is clear differentiation between the waking part of the room and the sleeping part. Angle the television away from the bed. Use partitions or arrange the furniture strategically. Don't eat or read in bed.

5. *Socialize.* If you are fortunate enough to have a companion at this stage of life, try to coordinate your schedules to enjoy one another's company. However, even an older couple needs the stimulation of other company besides what they get at home. Sticking around the house limits vital social interaction, and when a person is alone, the needs are more urgent still. There may be more of a tendency to nap or snack or watch TV, which can disrupt your daily (and nightly) rhythms. Visit a social club, volunteer, or go see family and friends. Go to a museum. Be creative with your awake time. And if at all possible *walk* there.

6. *Medications.* There are two things to be especially careful about concerning medications. First, when it comes to taking prescription drugs, talk to your doctor about their possible side effects on sleep. Second, do not try over-the-counter sleep aids without talking to your doctor. This includes melatonin. Some of these medicines contain antihistamines and may give you a hangover feeling or cause other side effects such as difficulty

urinating. Furthermore, your metabolism changes with age and the active ingredients in everything from coffee to Lipitor need a careful review in terms of potential interactions or side effects.

7. *Monitor your drinking and smoking.* Watch not just what you drink and smoke, but when. Some people think that if they have been drinking and smoking until old age, a few more years won't hurt them. However, not only do alcohol and tobacco constitute a long-term threat but they have very negative short-term effects on your health, particularly as it pertains to sleep. Alcohol must be avoided prior to sleep because it is a sedative that wears off in the night, causing insomnia and the need to urinate. In the case of tobacco, not only is nicotine a stimulant, which is the basis of its physiological appeal to begin with, but it disrupts your heart function and breathing in ways that increase the danger of stroke, heart attack, and other organ failure. Leaving aside cancer and emphysema for the moment, cigarettes can further diminish the oxygen richness of your blood by compounding airway swelling and aggravating sleep apnea.

8. *Get help when you need it.* If you worry about your sleep to the point of fear or anxiety, get help from your doctor or a sleep specialist.

9. *Limit your use of sleeping pills.* If you already use sleeping pills, use them only as directed by your doctor. If they "aren't working," go back to the doctor, don't raise your dosage on your own.

10. *Keep in touch with your doctor.* If something is very wrong in your life—not just your sleeping but in your *24-hour day*—tell your doctor. Don't wait for an emergency.

The elderly are one of the fastest growing populations in the world, and as their numbers increase, so will their effect they have on society. With all of the problems that the elderly must face when confronted with a world insensitive to their needs, adding a sleep disorder only causes further isolation and dysfunction. Illness of the mind and/or body can be severely exacerbated in the elderly when they are suffering from a sleep disorder. Treating the sleep disorder can quite often alleviate both day and night symptoms. If you are caring for an elderly person, and are worried that they might be suffering from a sleep disorder, speak to a physician about getting help. By taking an active role, you increase their chances of going from golden nights to golden years and your chances for the associated peace of mind.

Geriatric 24-Hour Sleep-Wake Diary

If you have noticed changes in your sleep patterns that you attribute to advancing age in accordance with the information in this chapter, or if you have a family member or friends whom you suspect of having such problems, the geriatric sleep diary is designed for you. You will find the sleep diary on pages 284–85 in the back of the book.

___

LOW GEAR—THE PROBLEMS OF SHIFT WORKERS

A night shift operator was told to report to the sleep center. A supervisor had seen him while his bus was stopped at a depot. His eyes were closed and while they were, the bus rolled several inches. The patient told me he was tired but not asleep.

I found him to be very well adjusted to night work after 20 years. His family and friends had adapted to the demands of his hours and helped him create a shift worker paradise. A nine-to-fiver couldn't have had a more satisfying existence. He had a perfect record and was anxious to get a clearance and get back to work.

He had a convincing explanation for being tired at the time of the incident. His sister was very ill and he had spent the whole day shepherding her through numerous doctor visits and tests. But he made a mistake. He hadn't realized that missing a day's sleep might be a problem. They got home late so he took a two-hour nap, showered, ate dinner, and went to work.

After the interview and examination we sat in the consultation room where I summarized my findings. I started by fully supporting the supervisor's concern and the recommendation to his medical officer for a sleep evaluation. Based on his history of snoring and the slight elongation of his soft palate, I agreed with the request for a full sleep study. The study during his usual day sleep showed very mild sleep apnea. The apnea was only present when he was in REM sleep and "supine"—on his back. We refer to this as supine-locked sleep apnea.

On first hearing the diagnosis he was almost inconsolable. He knew of others who had been diagnosed with sleep apnea and he was certain this meant he would lose his job. What would happen to his wife and children and several others in his extended family who depended on him?

First of all, we altered his habit of sleeping on his back using the "low-tech" tennis ball therapy described in Chapter 7. Then we documented a normal full sleep followed by a MSLT. The sleep study revealed no sleep apnea and the MSLT showed no awake-time sleepiness (see to page 56 in Chapter 4 for a discussion of the use of the MSLT). All the data pointed to the lost sleep on the day of the incident as a cause of the head nod.

He returned to the medical department with a summary of the findings and a note supporting his return to full duty. The medical officer then cleared him to return to work without restrictions.

However, he learned a lesson, namely, that he couldn't take even occasional liberties with the routine that he had forged for himself over a period of years. Night shift work is a physiologically demanding way to make a living, even for night owls.

His supervisors, meanwhile, had behaved correctly. It is not for them to make exceptions or overlook lapses in employee performance. They were alert, conscientious, and informed about the medical implications of what had been observed.

As Different as Night and Day

For many years, shift workers—those who work outside the confines of the traditional day—have been paid more than their nine-to-five counterparts. In part, they were being compensated for missing out on the satisfactions of participating in "normal" life. But is that all they were missing out on?

This is a very delicate question in a world where a 24/7 economy is taken for granted. Some night shift labor will always have to be done locally, such as policing, firefighting, and bus driving. Other night shift labor, such as manufacturing and data processing, is subject to steady international competition in other time zones around the globe.

As the World Turns

Jobs are not all we are outsourcing. In many cases, we are also outsourcing the sleep disorders that go with shift work. Shift work–related sleep disorder is a global phenomenon. As you have read in earlier chapters, some of the best research on sleep disorder is being done at universities around the world. They wouldn't be studying these problems if they weren't having them in those societies.

In India, for example, hundreds of thousands of jobs have been created at call centers for foreign businesses. Our daytime is their nighttime and that means that more Indians, men and women in approximately equal numbers, are working at night. With those jobs are coming the health problems associated with shift work. The list of complaints by those who work in these call centers would be familiar to shift workers everywhere.

Here in the United States we need our shift workers. An estimated 40 percent of the American workforce works mostly nonstandard hours—evenings, overnight, on rotating schedules, or on weekends. They are critical for distributing goods as well as making them, and for staffing hospitals, transit facilities, and other businesses. The numbers are increasing elsewhere, too. However, considering that about 70 percent of shift workers report difficulty sleeping and some sleepiness while working, we have to consider whether we are using this invaluable resource wisely and well, as we do with all other aspects of business. The fact is that the way we as a society manage our shift workers imposes tremendous economic costs.

What Are the Costs of Shift Work?

Circadian Technologies, a firm that advises companies on strategies for improving the efficiency of their shift workers, estimates the economic costs of poor shift management in the United States as follows:

Excess Cost*			
	To Operations	Per Employee	As a % of Total
Absenteeism	$50.4 billion	$2,102	24%
Lost Productivity	$79.4 billion	$3,309	39%
Turnover	$39.1 billion	$1,631	19%
Accidents	$8.5 billion	$354	4%
Health Care	$28.2 billion	$1,181	14%
Total	$205.6 billion	$8,577	100%

*Adapted from Circadian Technologies Web site: http://www.circadian.com/.

I am not going to argue economics here or give advice to management, either. What I am going to do is describe how shift work affects your health and help you develop individual strategies for maintaining your own health if you must continue to work after the rest of your community has retired for the night.

As described in Chapter 4, our sleeping patterns are largely inborn. Most of us have evolved to be active during the day and to rest at night. Our conquest of darkness probably began with the ability to start fires—Greek mythology says that the young god Prometheus brought fire from the heavens to mankind, and we now refer to great scientific breakthroughs as "Promethean." Certainly electricity qualifies as one of these.

But while fire and later electricity have changed the way people can shape their environment, that control doesn't extend to the body's circadian rhythms, which have evolved over thousands of years. Like the tides, our bodies still operate on a schedule that doesn't easily change just because we want it to.

Circadian Rhythms and Work

As discussed in Chapter 2, the sleep-wake cycle is controlled by several mind-body rhythms. The circadian synchronization is orchestrated by the SCN (suprachiasmastic nucleus in the brain), which receives input from light via the eyes. This sets the synchronization of the day-night clock described in the owl-lark chart in Chapter 4. The expression of the circadian clock gene is one of the factors that account for owl or lark behavior.

The Early Bird Gene

The first category of circadian-related sleep disorders is referred to as "endogenous." These arise when our inborn nature is out of synch with the working world. For some of us, our genetic programming is so powerful that we cannot adapt our schedule to the rest of the working world. In one family in Utah, for example, everyone falls asleep at 7 P.M. and awakens at 3–4 A.M. When their sleep-wake habits were studied, they were all found to have a unique gene thought to be responsible for the "extreme lark" behavior. No amount of conditioning can reset a genetically programmed circadian schedule so at odds with the general norm.

The family in Utah is an extreme case, but its basic lesson can be applied to all of us.

A second class of circadian sleep disorders are "behavioral." These arise when we try to impose an inappropriate schedule on ourselves. Weekend teenager syndrome is an example of a behavioral sleep disorder. As I sit here writing this chapter, my sons and their friends are brushing off the felt of a card table, preparing for a long night of entertainment. They will get up late tomorrow. When the group returns tomorrow night to try and win back their chips, the whole process will repeat itself. It's okay to challenge the body clock this way now and then. If we let this "extreme owl" behavior persist, however, after a while we will start to get calls from school pointing out that our kids are dozing in class.

What does learned sleep-wake behavior have to do with the workforce? It shows that people can accommodate themselves to unaccustomed hours only so much. You can "get used" to living this way to some extent, but for many, this behavior will clash with your true circadian rhythms and sleep needs. In that case, your work performance and quality of life will suffer.

The third class of circadian disorders are known as "temporal," or time shift, disorders; they stem from changes in your orientation to the clock and the rising and setting of the sun. Jet lag is an example of a temporal disorder, especially when traveling east across time zones: Say you leave New York for London this evening, eat, watch a movie, and, if you are lucky, sleep all in the space of six hours. And when you arrive in London the next day, it's rush hour. But you're just going through the motions. Your body is still on early morning sleep time and simply hasn't had enough time to do all the things it's supposed to do. Trips toward the west are generally tolerated better.

Some shift work sleep disorders are very much like jet lag, especially when you work rotating shifts. In jet lag and rotating shift work, light cues occur at different times from what our body expects. We have to perform accustomed functions at unaccustomed times. Mental and physical functions are best done according to established rhythms of an entire collection of hormonal, chemical, and organ systems. The brain is receiving environmental and behavioral signals to start the day when most of the body is getting ready for sleep. Shift workers do their best to synchronize their bodies' awake state and sleep tendencies with the demands of their jobs, but sometimes their bodies are playing musical chairs, and they don't stop when the music does. The result is subtle changes in their physical and mental health.

Physical Disease, Social Discord

Shift workers have an increased incidence of cardiovascular disease, gastrointestinal disorders, menstrual irregularities, weakened immunity, certain cancers, emotional problems, divorce, and social discord.

An article by two physicians, Leslie Olson and Antonio Ambrogetti, published in the *Medical Journal of Australia,* reported: "Nightshift workers seldom sleep more than five or six hours in each 24-hour period, so that after seven nights the accumulated sleep deficit is 15 to 20 hours." They estimated that it takes a minimum of 48 hours off to make up the difference, which can't be easy if the workers have any other demands on their time, such as spouses and children.

The shortfall takes the biggest bite out of REM sleep and stage-2 sleep. So not only does a midnight-to-eight worker suffer from minimal energy and alertness right in the middle of the "working day," but also suffers from chronic sleep deprivation because of poor-quality daytime sleep. No wonder, then, that many shift workers are obsessed with sleep.

Stomach Rumblings, GI Jitters?

The gastrointestinal tract suffers particularly from circadian disruption, as international travelers will tell you. You thought it was just the airline food that made your stomach hurt on that overnight flight to visit Uncle Seamus and Aunt Mollie in Dublin. Only partly. It was also the fact that you were eating it at your normal bedtime and trying to digest it when your body thought it should be sound asleep.

Digestion benefits greatly from regular mealtimes, trips to the bathroom, and rest. Shift workers' bowels suffer from "jet lag" especially those on variable schedules night after night. They are afflicted with an appetizing list of ailments such as constipation, diarrhea, excessive flatulence, abdominal pain, and heartburn at two to three times the rate of others. They have diets high in saturated fats because that's generally all that is available late at night, or they rely on vending machine fare. They eat too much fast food after work because they're too tired to cook for themselves. "Lunch" can be a terrible problem. Their digestion goes to sleep just before they eat that late-night cheeseburger, and it will just sit there. Combine this with extra coffee drinking, smoking, and psychological stress, and you've got the basis of true misery.

Given their eating habits, and other factors, rotating shift workers are also at higher risk of heart disease, 40 to 50 percent higher, according to the Helsinki Heart Study of the Finnish population, which was conducted over a five-year period. A study of female shift workers showed that American nurses who worked rotating shifts for six years or more had a 51 percent higher coronary heart disease risk than day nurses.

Researchers Find Fat Deposits in Antarctica

Scientists who work in Antarctica are there to serve the cause of human knowledge, but they also make a unique population for the study of human physiology.

Researchers from the University of Surrey in Guildford, England, studied 12 healthy night shift workers aged 24 to 34 years at the British Antarctic Survey station at Halley Bay in Antarctica.

They measured hormonal and metabolic responses to meals during daytime on normal working days, at night at the beginning of a period of night shift work, and during the day when the workers went back from night shifts to days. They also checked blood and urine.

The researchers found that after meals, blood levels of glucose, insulin, and triacylglycerol (TAG), one of the fats that can store energy, were significantly higher among night shift workers than in normal daytime hours. Furthermore, while levels of glucose and insulin returned to preshift levels two days after workers returned to day shifts, TAG levels remained elevated. TAG levels are measured periodically by your doctor and are one of the key factors in the formation of fat deposits on the inside of arteries. This is one component of the mechanism that leads to vascular and heart disease.

Can't We Reset Our Body Clocks?

But can't we catch up? Can't we readjust our body clocks so that the time we work and the time we sleep don't matter? Drs. Olson and Ambrogetti have their strong doubts. In their *Medical Journal of Australia* article, they say: "Physiological adaptation to night work is largely a myth and there is no reason to extend periods of night work in the hope that adaptation will occur. For intellectually demanding tasks, short periods of night work (one or two shifts) are better tolerated than longer periods because the accumulated sleep deficit is less. It is easy to demonstrate that the progressive sleep loss of a seven-night roster causes a progressive rise in accidents and a fall in productivity." The consequences are well known. Concentration, the ability to process new information, and short-term memory all suffer. Performance becomes erratic.

Many of us have what doctors call "clinical intolerance" of night shift work. In short, we never adapt. Moreover, even those who are tolerant at a younger age seem to become intolerant between the ages of 40 and 50.

In addition to the physiological effects of this reversal, daytime sleepers develop many behaviors to compensate. They take drugs—stimulants or coffee to stay up and alcohol or sedatives to rest. Also, noise and light, even if they don't fully awaken someone, will register with the daytime sleeper and alter the sleep cycles.

Hearts That Work Nights

A study published several years ago by scientists at the University of Milan detailed the heart problems of male steelworkers who worked three shifts—6 A.M.–2 P.M., 2–10 P.M., and 10 P.M.–6 A.M. Their shifts were rotated weekly. The workers were given two days to adjust each time they changed shifts, and then ECG recordings were monitored continuously for a 24-hour period, and they were subject to a battery of other cardiac tests. The researchers found that regardless of work schedule, the chemical and nerve activity that determine the level of heart function remained on a daytime schedule. Levels rose during the day and subsided at night. What this suggests is that the heart is programmed to function according to its circadian timetable, regardless of what we are telling our bodies to do.

Dr. Raffaello Furlan, who headed the team at the University of Milan, said, "This resistance of the body's internal clock to change with varied work schedules indicates that people don't adapt as easily as we think to shift work, and could explain why shift workers are at higher risk [of heart disease]."

The strain on the heart could be compared to trying to do vigorous exercise with muscles that can, in effect, never warm up. In addition, when workers have reduced levels of temperature and plasma cortisol, which are also programmed according to circadian rhythms, they will feel sleepy and less alert than they should be, and thus more prone to errors and accidents.

Social Life Plays Hard to Get

So the arithmetic of the 24-hour day is already stacked against the shift worker. Add to this the demands of family and friends, the traffic noises, the jet flights overhead, and the worker is really in a tough position. Twenty percent of shift workers are single mothers, who have to juggle child care arrangements. Couples in which one spouse works a nonstandard shift are more likely to have family and marital problems. Shift work is a way of life—not always a voluntary one—yet the world makes few concessions to it.

The health effects are disturbing. Parents give up sleep in order to be with their children. They are also subject to more menstrual irregularities, colds, flu, and weight gain than day workers.

No Legal Recourse

In 1999, the U.S. Supreme Court refused to hear an appeal by a radio newscaster named William Scheffler, who was fired and denied long-term disability payments for health problems he claimed were caused by continual changes in his schedule required by his employer.

After working in Princeton for a radio news service for several years, he got a new job that would require filling in for other newscasters, which was fine as long as the service didn't broadcast overnight. When they went to a 24-hour-a-day format, his schedule changed as often as three or four times a week, including night shifts, hours that he said "were not in his job description." He claimed there had been 60 shift changes in 1994. That was the year he began suffering from medical problems including high blood pressure, irregular heartbeat, and migraine headaches. He fell asleep while driving and had an accident. These problems are now known as "shift work sleep disorder."

After failing to reach a desired accommodation with his employer, he was fired. He later sued under provisions of the Americans with Disabilities Act. However, he lost in federal district court and in the court of appeals, and the Supreme Court has let the ruling stand, denying him further legal recourse.

Nurses

It doesn't take a doctor to know that nurses are among our most vital members of the night shift workforce. Not surprisingly, the profession pays a good deal of attention to the needs of its members, including their sleep needs. In *RN* magazine, Barbara Weiss recommends the following as part of a "night shift survival guide."

- Sleep and eat well before your shift.
- Eat balanced meals, with complex carbohydrates combined with some protein and moderate amounts of fat.
- Wear a digital 24-hour watch to keep from being disoriented about night or day.
- Eat or drink something warm if hormonal changes make you feel especially chilled.

Shift Work Life Doesn't Have to Be Hell

I am an avid golfer but I don't get to play as much as I would like. I frequently get up way too early in the morning when tee times are available on short notice. On those occasions, I am often given an object lesson in the fact that night work suits some people just fine. I run into people whose night owl circadian rhythms have steered them into a suitable career choice, but who love golf. Thus, they are able to go straight from work to the golf course and they can do it several times a week, where I have to drag myself out of bed to do it.

Moreover, in families where one parent works days and the other works nights, children can have an advantage that is rare enough in two-earner households. If the whole family is organized to make sure that both parents get enough sleep, the children can have a parent on call for more of the day than they would if both parents work days.

Whether night work agrees with you or doesn't, there are strategies that can help you make the most of the available time.

The Evaluation of Shift Workers' Sleep Complaints

We see a large number of shift workers at our center and evaluate them using a combination of detailed medical and sleep history, which helps identify all possible causes of sleep disorders. We also use standard sleep questionnaires and screening tools to help identify sleep apnea, leg movement disorders, poor sleep hygiene, insomnia, medical or psychiatric illness, and neurologic disorders including narcolepsy. In other words, the first order of the day is not to miss a specific sleep disorder or condition causing a sleep disorder by assuming that the patient's complaint is due solely to shift work.

If a sleep disorder is suspected, the sleep study will be performed as close to the scheduled sleep time as possible, day or night. This may also be followed by an MSLT (multiple sleep latency test), again coinciding with the patients' wake time and immediately following the sleep study. A patient-completed sleep diary may also help evaluate the quantity and quality of sleep. (Refer to the shift workers diary in the diary section on pages 286–87 in the back of the book.)

ACTIGRAPHY

An additional tool, used usually in research, looks at the worker's motion and lack of motion over several weeks. This is called actigraphy.

Keeping an electronic log of the way patients move during the entire day and week can also help uncover sleep-wake dysfunction in shift workers. Actigraphy records activity during waking and sleeping without application of any electrodes. It consists of a movement detector—the most popular one is worn as a watch—and has considerable memory, so it can record when you move and when you are still, as in sleep, including periods of dozing when you should be working. Data is plotted against time for a week or two and the results are downloaded for review. The patient can wear it continuously as he or she goes about routine daily activities. Actigraphy is ideal for extended examination of the sleep-wake cycle in shift workers and in the patient's home environment.

There is a very close correlation, up to 90 percent, between the rest-activity findings recorded by the actigraph and the sleep-wake pattern as determined by an overnight sleep study. This information may help identify poor sleep patterns or insufficient sleep and guide in scheduling future shift work schedules.

Treatment Options

LOOKING FOR SYMPTOMS

A study of healthy adults age 20–38 showed the effects of minimal sleep loss over a two-week period. The deficit was cumulative and this sleep debt had substantial effects on memory, alertness, and overall performance. The patient was for the most part unaware of the subtle initial changes.

Since the signs may be subtle and people are very adaptable, medical practitioners should screen with a series of questions looking for these symptoms:

- Uncontrollable or unintentional sleep episodes
- Lack of focus or lapses in attention
- Decreased performance at work or home
- Increase in job, home, or traffic accidents
- Increase or change in nap patterns at home or on the job
- Unexplained difficulty treating a medical or mental illness

Recognizing these signs may be your first step in preventing a more serious and chronic condition.

INDIVIDUAL STRATEGIES FOR A BETTER LIFE ON SHIFT WORK

Get the most out of the sleep you get. Follow good sleep hygiene rules established for non–shift workers. This includes avoiding excess caffeine and nicotine and making the sleep environment quiet, dark, and comfortable. As we have seen, managing one's life for sleep also entails managing the waking life. Vigorous exercise is an important component of waking life, but it shouldn't be done too close to bedtime; this will allow the hormonal and metabolic processes to achieve levels conducive to sleep. This is as true for night shift workers as it is for daytime workers, so exercise will have to be timed accordingly.

Meals are another factor. As with day workers, large meals shouldn't be consumed too close to bedtime after a night shift. Night workers are also at a disadvantage socially compared with day workers. If at all possible, it is advisable to schedule meals with other members of the family or with friends so as not to lose touch with their world, even if supper is really breakfast.

Educate your family and friends. Don't try to live in both worlds at the same time. Let your loved ones know how important your sleep time is. Get an answering machine and leave the phone unplugged in your bedroom.

Sleep in split periods. If you cannot get a continuous sleep, split sleep is better than no sleep. It entails three to four hours of sleep immediately before work and three to four hours immediately afterward. This has the advantage that at least part of each day's sleep falls when it is dark, the time when the body "expects" to sleep.

Use anchor sleep. Anchor sleep is a technique used following one's shift during a series of nights. It is basically an alternative to switching to a diurnal ("of the day"—the opposite of "nocturnal") orientation. Switching to a diurnal schedule for weekends only, for example, should be avoided.

An example of anchor sleep would be staying up until 2 or 3 A.M. and then sleeping until 10 or 11 A.M. That way the shift worker gets some time to socialize as diurnal people do but doesn't completely lose a nocturnal orientation.

Scrap random naps. Naps can create big problems. While regularly scheduled naps can be effective, and some industries with multiple workers on night shifts include them in their shift design, in general, random naps can make your regular sleeping program less effective. Routine is important to the quality of sleep whatever schedule you work on, and 40 winks here and 40 winks there can make it harder to get sleep during the planned sleep period without increasing your alertness level or improving your mood.

That said, however, a short nap before the ride home may be a lifesaver. In a 1999 National Sleep Foundation poll of those who work "extended hours", 41 percent reported that they had dozed at the wheel, compared with 28 percent of day workers. The NSF recommends car-pooling or taking public transportation, if practical.

Medication can also be considered but only after a thorough evaluation and workup by a doctor experienced in sleep medicine.

Hypnotics and Alcohol

Hypnotics—sleeping pills—should not be routinely used by night workers. Occasionally they are useful for short-term treatment of some acute insomnias. However, while they do increase total sleep time during the day, they do not hasten resetting of rhythms to night shifts or improve alertness during the night. When used, they should be short-acting in order to avoid residual effects during work. Benzodiazepines should also be avoided for similar reasons.

Alcohol may help you get to sleep but the sleep is of a terrible quality. It reduces REM sleep, which is already in short supply during daytime sleep anyway. When the alcohol is metabolized, you wake up and suffer the frustration of poor sleep. Over time the effects of chronic alcohol use will cause more than a sleep disorder.

Stimulants

Many shift workers rely on caffeine. However, while it can increase alertness, it should not be consumed within four hours of a planned sleep period.

Of all the available amphetamines, amphetamine-like substances, and newer medications termed "CNS alerting drugs," Modafinil, aka Provigil, is both the safest and most effective. It was recently approved for use with shift workers with excessive daytime or wake-time sleepiness. The biggest challenge will be when, how long, and how often it should be used.

Antidepressants

There is little evidence to support use of antidepressants for shift work sleep disorders, although each person must be evaluated for other conditions that might benefit from their use.

One pharmacological agent that holds promise for moving the sleep phase in the needed direction is melatonin. This is a hormone secreted nightly by the pineal gland in response to darkness. Melatonin when used optimally has a sedating effect but, more important, has been shown to hasten resetting of circadian rhythms in certain circumstances. Studies are currently under way on the use of melatonin for shift workers to help them make the transition from one schedule to another.

Bright light therapy, discussed in detail in Chapter 14, can also hasten resetting of circadian rhythms. Lights can increase alertness on the night shift and rapidly convert circadian rhythms; while in the early morning (5 to 7 A.M.) they can hasten adaptation back to days.

Exercise is a useful strategy for adapting to shift work. Not only does it improve general mood, but it also promotes alertness on night shift (if not too strenuous). It has been shown to increase circadian adaptation as well. Aerobic exercise done immediately after awakening is most effective, no matter which shift you work.

If you have continued difficulty initiating sleep or staying asleep, tell your doctor. Shift workers can develop other sleep disorders or other medical problems just like anyone else and symptoms should not automatically be attributed to shift work, especially if they persist or get worse.

Tips for Employers

- Proper lighting, adequate ventilation, and comfortable temperatures contribute to safety and greater productivity.
- A spacious, comfortable, and clean dining area that serves nutritious food will offer a break from fast food and limited social interaction.
- Stock the vending machines with something more nutritious than candy bars and chips.
- Many employers are offering nap rooms or pods.
- Provide exercise with adequate space and exercise equipment and time to use them.
- Offer educational counseling and support groups.
- Outside consultants can help develop scheduling, rest, and nutrition strategies for groups of employees with complicated or high-risk jobs.

There's No Turning Back

We need our shift workers to be healthy and happy. It is no surprise that keeping a regular circadian-like schedule is one of the keys to minimizing shift work–related illness, and that an unpredictable, variable shift is most harmful. There is some irony in the fact that the advanced technologies that push us to more shift work remind us of our physical limitations. Medications are at times lifesaving, although, there is no improving on the natural order of our day to night existence.

As we move closer to the development of more effective sleep-wake neurochemicals, we will be faced with the challenge of how to use them wisely. What will the prescription read? Here's a thought: "℞ Take one to sleep well and one to work well, and both to live well. Use in conjunction with good diet and exercise. Refill only as needed for a better life."

SLEEP DIARIES

The following are sleep diaries for specific groups discussed in this book. Each has been adapted from standard formats specifically for *Sleep to Save Your Life*. The information compiled in the appropriate diary for you or for a loved one will provide you and your doctor with the information needed to begin to make a change for the better in health and quality of life. It is recommended that you make enlarged copies for easier reading and data entry, and where a two-week diary is indicated, make two copies. You may also find these at the Web site: www.SleeptoSaveYourLife.com.

SLEEP

	Time to bed	Time it took to fall asleep	Number of times you woke up	Time you woke up	Time you got out of bed	How you felt when you first woke up
Day 1 Date____ Day____	PM_____ AM_____	Minutes____ Hours____	Woke during the night __times	PM_____ AM_____	PM_____ AM_____	Well rested____ Slightly rested__ Not rested____
Day 2 Date____ Day____	PM_____ AM_____	Minutes____ Hours____	Woke during the night __times	PM_____ AM_____	PM_____ AM_____	Well rested____ slightly rested__ not rested____
Day 3 Date____ Day____	PM_____ AM_____	Minutes____ Hours____	Woke during the night __times	PM_____ AM_____	PM_____ AM_____	Well rested____ slightly rested__ not rested____
Day 4 Date____ Day____	PM_____ AM_____	Minutes____ Hours____	Woke during the night __times	PM_____ AM_____	PM_____ AM_____	Well rested____ slightly rested__ not rested____
Day 5 Date____ Day____	PM_____ AM_____	Minutes____ Hours____	Woke during the night __times	PM_____ AM_____	PM_____ AM_____	Well rested____ slightly rested__ not rested____
Day 6 Date____ Day____	PM_____ AM_____	Minutes____ Hours____	Woke during the night __times	PM_____ AM_____	PM_____ AM_____	Well rested____ slightly rested__ not rested____
Day 7 Date____ Day____	PM_____ AM_____	Minutes____ Hours____	Woke during the night __times	PM_____ AM_____	PM_____ AM_____	Well rested____ slightly rested__ not rested____

◀ complete in the morning

WAKE DIARY

AND   WAKE

Total hours sleep	Briefly describe your sleep, including any problems.	Diet	Describe exercise time and duration.	Briefly describe your day, including naps or major stresses.	List your medication and times you take it.	Describe your bedtime routine.
Hours____		Number or amount of: Caffeine____ Alcohol____ Meals____				
Hours____		Number or amount of: Caffeine____ Alcohol____ Meals____				
Hours____		Number or amount of: Caffeine____ Alcohol____ Meals____				
Hours____		Number or amount of: Caffeine____ Alcohol____ Meals____				
Hours____		Number or amount of: Caffeine____ Alcohol____ Meals____				
Hours____		Number or amount of: Caffeine____ Alcohol____ Meals____				
Hours____		Number or amount of: Caffeine____ Alcohol____ Meals____				

←   ← complete before bed →   →

Use the back of this page to expand on any question

SLEEP

	Describe the bedtime routine.	Time to bed	Time it took to fall asleep	Number of times you woke up during the night	Time you woke up	Time you got out of bed	How you felt when you first woke up
Day 1 Date_____ Day_____		PM_____ AM_____	Minutes_____ Hours_____	During the night woke _____times	PM_____ AM_____	PM_____ AM_____	Well rested_____ Slightly rested_____ Not rested_____
Day 2 Date_____ Day_____		PM_____ AM_____	Minutes_____ Hours_____	During the night woke _____times	PM_____ AM_____	PM_____ AM_____	Well rested_____ Slightly rested_____ Not rested_____
Day 3 Date_____ Day_____		PM_____ AM_____	Minutes_____ Hours_____	During the night woke _____times	PM_____ AM_____	PM_____ AM_____	Well rested_____ Slightly rested_____ Not rested_____
Day 4 Date_____ Day_____		PM_____ AM_____	Minutes_____ Hours_____	During the night woke _____times	PM_____ AM_____	PM_____ AM_____	Well rested_____ Slightly rested_____ Not rested_____
Day 5 Date_____ Day_____		PM_____ AM_____	Minutes_____ Hours_____	During the night woke _____times	PM_____ AM_____	PM_____ AM_____	Well rested_____ Slightly rested_____ Not rested_____
Day 6 Date_____ Day_____		PM_____ AM_____	Minutes_____ Hours_____	During the night woke _____times	PM_____ AM_____	PM_____ AM_____	Well rested_____ Slightly rested_____ Not rested_____
Day 7 Date_____ Day_____		PM_____ AM_____	Minutes_____ Hours_____	During the night woke _____times	PM_____ AM_____	PM_____ AM_____	Well rested_____ Slightly rested_____ Not rested_____

◄———————— complete in the morning ————————

**Parents or guardians should complete the diary by asking questions or by direct observation.

DIARY FOR CHILDREN**

AND   WAKE

Total hours sleep	Briefly describe your sleep, including any problems.	Diet: List the number or amount	Time spent in hours	Describe excerise time and duration	List your medication and times you take it.	Briefly describe your day, including naps, energy level, or other problems.
____ Hours		Cups of soda___ juice___ water___ Caffeine____ Meals____ Snacks_____	School___ TV___ Video games___ Reading___ Web___			
____ Hours		Cups of soda___ juice___ water___ Caffeine____ Meals____ Snacks_____	School___ TV___ Video games___ Reading___ Web___			
____ Hours		Cups of soda___ juice___ water___ Caffeine____ Meals____ Snacks_____	School___ TV___ Video games___ Reading___ Web___			
____ Hours		Cups of soda___ juice___ water___ Caffeine____ Meals____ Snacks_____	School___ TV___ Video games___ Reading___ Web___			
____ Hours		Cups of soda___ juice___ water___ Caffeine____ Meals____ Snacks_____	School___ TV___ Video games___ Reading___ Web___			
____ Hours		Cups of soda___ juice___ water___ Caffeine____ Meals____ Snacks_____	School___ TV___ Video games___ Reading___ Web___			
____ Hours		Cups of soda___ juice___ water___ Caffeine____ Meals____ Snacks_____	School___ TV___ Video games___ Reading___ Web___			

→   ←— complete before bed —→

Use the back of this page to expand on any question

GERIATRIC SLEEP

A time to bed
B you first fell asleep
C asleep (includes naps)
D woke from sleep briefly (i.e., bathroom or noise)
E prolonged awakening after sleep
F first awake after sleep

Use the legend above to fill in the 24-hour sleep diary. Each small box is 30 minutes.

Time	PM 6		7		8		9		10		11		mid-night 12		1		2		3		4		5		6	
Example	I		N	N	N	C	C			N	N	P		A	B	C	C	C	C	D	C	F	E	E	E	E	G
Day 1 Date__ Day__																											
Day 2 Date__ Day____																											
Day 3 Date__ Day____																											
Day 4 Date__ Day_____																											
Day 5 Date__ Day____																											
Day 6 Date__ Day_____																											
Day 7 Date__ Day____																											

**To be completed by the patient, guardian, or caregiver.

Briefly describe the average or typical sleep:

Briefly describe the time spent when not sleeping:

-WAKE DIARY**

- G when you first get out of bed
- H drank caffeine
- I ate a meal or snack
- J workout or exercise including walks
- K housekeeping or similar activity
- L shopping or other activity outside the home

- M socializing
- N watched TV or similar activity
- O reading
- P drank alcohol
- Q performed a routine before bed
- X screaming, shouting, or agitated behavior

				noon							Refreshed from sleep 1 = very 2 = moderate 3 = not	Number of hours you slept	Describe your sleep.
7	8	9	10	11	12	1	2	3	4	5			
H I	N N	N I	H		I		N N N N		C C C		1	5	restless
												___ Hours	
												___ Hours	
												___ Hours	
												___ Hours	
												___ Hours	
												___ Hours	
												___ Hours	

	Briefly describe your shift.	Time of meals	Number or amount of:	Time of excerise	Number of times I thought about sleep	Productivity level at work	Things done for self
Day 1 Date____ Day____		AM____ PM____ AM____ PM____	Caffeine____ Alcohol____ Medication____	AM____ PM____ AM____ PM____	a few____ several____ many____ all day____	high____ mod____ low____	hobbies____ visited friends____ other____
Day 2 Date____ Day____		AM____ PM____ AM____ PM____	Caffeine____ Alcohol____ Medication____	AM____ PM____ AM____ PM____	a few____ several____ many____ all day____	high____ mod____ low____	hobbies____ visited friends____ other____
Day 3 Date____ Day____		AM____ PM____ AM____ PM____	Caffeine____ Alcohol____ Medication____	AM____ PM____ AM____ PM____	a few____ several____ many____ all day____	high____ mod____ low____	hobbies____ visited friends____ other____
Day 4 Date____ Day____		AM____ PM____ AM____ PM____	Caffeine____ Alcohol____ Medication____	AM____ PM____ AM____ PM____	a few____ several____ many____ all day____	high____ mod____ low____	hobbies____ visited friends____ other____
Day 5 Date____ Day____		AM____ PM____ AM____ PM____	Caffeine____ Alcohol____ Medication____	AM____ PM____ AM____ PM____	a few____ several____ many____ all day____	high____ mod____ low____	hobbies____ visited friends____ other____
Day 6 Date____ Day____		AM____ PM____ AM____ PM____	Caffeine____ Alcohol____ Medication____	AM____ PM____ AM____ PM____	a few____ several____ many____ all day____	high____ mod____ low____	hobbies____ visited friends____ other____
Day 7 Date____ Day____		AM____ PM____ AM____ PM____	Caffeine____ Alcohol____ Medication____	AM____ PM____ AM____ PM____	a few____ several____ many____ all day____	high____ mod____ low____	hobbies____ visited friends____ other____

◄──── complete at the end of the wake period before sleep ────

7-DAY SLEEP-WAKE DIARY

			SLEEP						
Things done for others	Naps: Time and duration	At the end of the workday, I felt:	Time to bed	Time it took to fall asleep	Number of times I woke up	Time I woke up	Time I got out of bed	Total hours I slept	Briefly describe your sleep.
a few____ several____ many____ all day____	Time/hours ____/____ ____/____	tired____ rested____ neither____	AM ____ PM	Mins ____ Hrs	1 2 3 4 5 6 7 other ____	PM ____ AM	PM ____ AM	____ Hrs	
a few____ several____ many____ all day____	Time/hours ____/____ ____/____	tired____ rested____ neither____	AM ____ PM	Mins ____ Hrs	1 2 3 4 5 6 7 other ____	PM ____ AM	PM ____ AM	____ Hrs	
a few____ several____ many____ all day____	Time/hours ____/____ ____/____	tired____ rested____ neither____	AM ____ PM	Mins ____ Hrs	1 2 3 4 5 6 7 other ____	PM ____ AM	PM ____ AM	____ Hrs	
a few____ several____ many____ all day____	Time/hours ____/____ ____/____	tired____ rested____ neither____	AM ____ PM	Mins ____ Hrs	1 2 3 4 5 6 7 other ____	PM ____ AM	PM ____ AM	____ Hrs	
a few____ several____ many____ all day____	Time/hours ____/____ ____/____	tired____ rested____ neither____	AM ____ PM	Mins ____ Hrs	1 2 3 4 5 6 7 other ____	PM ____ AM	PM ____ AM	____ Hrs	
a few____ several____ many____ all day____	Time/hours ____/____ ____/____	tired____ rested____ neither____	AM ____ PM	Mins ____ Hrs	1 2 3 4 5 6 7 other ____	PM ____ AM	PM ____ AM	____ Hrs	
a few____ several____ many____ all day____	Time/hours ____/____ ____/____	tired____ rested____ neither____	AM ____ PM	Mins ____ Hrs	1 2 3 4 5 6 7 other ____	PM ____ AM	PM ____ AM	____ Hrs	

⟶   ⟵ complete after sleep period ⟶

Use the back of this page to expand on any question

Peppard, P. E. et al. Prospective Study of the Association between Sleep-Disordered Breathing and Hypertension. *New England Journal of Medicine* 342, no. 19 (2000): 1378–84.

Lacasse, Y., C. Godbout, and F. Sériès. "Health-Related Quality of Life in Obstructive Sleep Apnea." *European Respiration Journal* 19 (2002): 494–503.

Peker, Y., J. Hedner, J. Norum, and H. Kraiczi. Increased Incidence of Cardiovascular Disease in Middle-Aged Men with Obstructive Sleep Apnea: A 7-Year Follow-Up. *American Journal of Respiratory Critical Care Medicine* 166, no. 2 (July 15, 2002): 159–65.

Harbison, Joseph, Philip O'Reilly, and Walter T. McNicholas. "Cardiac Rhythm Disturbances in the Obstructive Sleep Apnea Syndrome Effects of Nasal Continuous Positive Airway Pressure Therapy." *Chest* 118 (2000): 591–95.

Becker, Heinrich F., A. Jerrentrup, T. Ploch, Ludger Grote, Thomas Penzel, Colin E. Sullivan, and Peter Hermann. "Effect of Nasal Continuous Positive Airway Pressure Treatment on Blood Pressure in Patients with Obstructive Sleep Apnea." *Circulation* 107 (2003): 68.

Meslier, N., F. Gagnadoux, P. Giraud, C. Person, H. Ouksel, T. Urban, and J.-L. Racineux. "Impaired Glucose-Insulin Metabolism in Males with Obstructive Sleep Apnea Syndrome." *European Respiration Journal* 22 (2003): 156–60.

Nasseem, S., B. Chaudhary, and N. Collop. "Attention Deficit Hyperactivity Disorder in Adults and Obstructive Sleep Apnea." *Chest* 119, no. 1 (2001): 294–96.

"Sleep Disorder Linked to Depression." BBC Online, Friday, March 1, 2002. Available from: http://news.bbc.co.uk/2/hi/health/1846845.stm.

Curry, Pat. "Too Sleepy for Sex?" *Health Scout News,* September 16, 2003. Available from: http://preventdisease.com/news/articles/too_sleepy_for_sex.shtml.

CHAPTER 8: NARCOLEPSY—WHEN SLEEP "ATTACKS"

Beusterien, K. M., A. E. Rogers, J. A. Walsleben, et al. "Health-Related Quality of Life Effects of Modafinil for Treatment of Narcolepsy." *Sleep* 22 (1999): 757–65.

Adapted from Cerner Multum, Inc. Version: 1.03. Revision date February 13, 2004.

CHAPTER 9: RESTLESS LEGS—PAIN IN MOTION

Walters, Arthur S. The International Restless Legs Syndrome Study. "Towards a Better Definition of the Restless Legs Syndrome." *Movement Disorders* 10 (1995): 634–43.

O'Connor, Anahad. "Restless Legs: Uncomfortable and Overlooked." *The New York Times,* May 25, 2004.

Sevim, S., O. Dogu, H. Kaleagasi, M. Aral, O. Metin, and H. Çamdeviren. "Correlation of Anxiety and Depression Symptoms in Patients with Restless Legs Syndrome: A Population Based Survey." *Journal of Neurology, Neurosurgery, and Psychiatry* 75 (2004): 226–30.

Chokroverty S., and J. Jankovic. "Restless Legs Syndrome. A Disease in Search of Identity." *Neurology* 52 (1999): 907–10.

Montplaisir, J., S. Boucher, G. Poirier, G. Lavigne, O. Lapierre, and P. Lesperance. "Clinical, Polysomnographic, and Genetic Characteristics of Restless Legs Syndrome: A Study of 133 Patients Diagnosed with New Standard Criteria. *Movement Disorders* 12 (1997): 61–65.

CHAPTER 10: INSOMNIA

Morin, Charles M. *Insomnia: Psychological Assessment and Management.* New York: Guilford, 1993.

Boehmer, Lisa N., Joshi John, Jerome M. Siegel, and Ming-Fung Wu. "Cataplexy-Active Neurons in the Hypothalamus: Implications for the Role of Histamine in Sleep and Waking Behavior." *Neuron* 42 (May 27, 2004): 619–34.

Harris, Louis. *Sleeplessness, Pain and the Workplace.* A report prepared by Louis Harris & Associates, Inc., for the National Sleep Foundation. Washington, D.C.: 1997.

Walsh, J. K. and C. L. Engelhardt. "The Direct Economic Costs of Insomnia in the United States for 1995." *Sleep* 22, suppl. 2 (May 1, 1999): S386–93.

Kryger, M. H., T. Roth, and W. C. Dement (eds.), *Principles and Practice of Sleep Medicine.* Philadelphia: Saunders, 1994.

Chesson, A. L., W. M. Anderson, M. Littner, et al. "Practice Parameters for the Nonpharmacologic Treatment of Chronic Insomnia." An American Academy of Sleep Medicine report. *Standards of Practice Committee of the American Academy of Sleep Medicine.* In *Sleep* 22, no. 8 (December 15, 1999): 1128–33.

Czeisler, C. A., C. Cajochen, and F. W. Turek. "Melatonin in the Regulation of Sleep and Circadian Rhythms. In *Principles and Practice of Sleep Medicine,* edited by M. H. Kryger, T. Ruth, and W. C. Dement. New York: McGraw-Hill (2000): 400–406.

Hauri, P. "Primary Insomnia." In *Principles and Practice of Sleep Medicine,* edited by M. H. Kryger, T. Roth, and W. C. Dement. New York: McGraw-Hill (2000): 633–39.

Roehrs, T., F. J. Zorick, and T. Roth. Transient and Short-term Insomnias. In *Principles and Practice of Sleep Medicine,* edited by M. H. Kryger, T. Roth, and W. C. Dement. New York: McGraw-Hill (2000): 624–32.

CHAPTER 11: "AROUND SLEEP"—THE MYSTERIES OF
PARASOMNIAS

Hurwitz, T.D., M.W. Mahowald, C.H. Schenck, et al. A Retrospective Out-
come Study and Review of Hypnosis as Treatment of Adults with Sleepwalking and Sleep Terror. *Journal of Nervous and Mental Disease* 179, no. 4
(April 1991): 228–33.

Thorpy, M.J. and P.B. Glovinsky. Parasomnias. *Psychiatric Clinics of North
America* 10, no.4 (Dec. 1987): 623–39.

Mahowald M.W. and C.H. Schenck. "Diagnosis and Management of Parasomnias. *Clinical Cornerstone* 2, no. 5 (2000): 48–57.

Willis, L. and J. Garcia. "Parasomnias: Epidemiology and Management. *Central Nervous System Drugs* 16, no. 12 (2002): 803–10.

CHAPTER 12: "WHAT'S THE MATTER WITH KIDS TODAY?"

2004 Sleep in America Poll. National Sleep Foundation. Available from:
http://www.sleepfoundation.org/2004poll.cfm.

Nieminen, Peter, Tuija Löppönen, Uolevi Tolonen, Peter Lanning, Mikael
Knip, and Heikki Löppönen. "Growth and Biochemical Markers of
Growth in Children with Snoring and Obstructive Sleep Apnea." *Pedi-
atrics* 109 (2002): e55.

O'Brien, Louise M., Cheryl R. Holbrook, Carolyn B. Mervis, Carrie J. Klaus,
Jennifer L. Bruner, Troy J. Raffield, Jennifer Rutherford, Rochelle C. Mehl,
Mei Wang, Andrew Tuell, Brittany C. Hume, and David Gozal. "Sleep
and Neurobehavioral Characteristics of 5- to 7-Year-Old Children with
Parentally Reported Symptoms of Attention-Deficit/Hyperactivity Disor-
der." *Pediatrics* 111 (2003): 554–63.

Tarasiuk, Ariel, Tzahit Simon, Asher Tal, and Haim Reuveni. "Adenotonsillectomy in Children with Obstructive Sleep Apnea Syndrome Reduces
Health Care Utilization." *Pediatrics* 113, no. 2 (February 2004): 351–56.

Golbin, A. et al. "Perennial Allergic Rhinitis (PAR) Increases Sleep Disorder
in Children." *Annals of Allergy* 68 (1992): 85.

Settipane R.A. "Complications of Allergic Rhinitis." *Allergy Asthma Proceedings* 20, no. 4 (July–August 1999): 209–13.

McColley S.A., J.L. Carroll, S. Curtis, et al. "High Prevalence of Allergic
Sensitization in Children with Habitual Snoring and Obstructive Sleep
Apnea." *Chest* 111 (1997): 170–73.

McLoughlin, J. et al. "The Realtionship of Allergies and Allergy Treatment to
School Performance and Student Behavior." *Annals of Allergy* 51 (1983):
506–10.

CHAPTER 13: UNIQUE CHANGES—WOMEN AND SLEEP

1998 Sleep in America Poll. National Sleep Foundation. Available
from:http://www.sleepfoundation.org/publications/1998poll.cfm.

Zhu, Jin Liang, Niels H. Hjollund, and Jorn Olsen. "Shift work, Duration of Pregnancy, and Birth Weight: The National Birth Cohort in Denmark." *American Journal of Obstetrics and Gynecology* 191, no. 1 (July 2004): 285–91.

2002 Sleep in America Poll. National Sleep Foundation. Available from: http://www.sleepfoundation.org/2002poll.cfm.

Kahneman, Daniel, Alan B. Krueger, David A. Schkade, Norbert Schwarz, and Arthur A. Stone. "A Survey Method for Characterizing Daily Life Experience: The Day Reconstruction Method." *Science* 306, no. 5702 (December 2004): 1776–80.

CHAPTER 14: OLDER, WISER, AND SLEEPIER

Census Bureau Information on Older Americans. Web site. Available from: http://www.heaton.org/census.htm.

Foley, D.J., A.A. Monjan, S.L. Brown, E.M. Simonsick, R.B. Wallace, and D.G. Blazer. "Sleep Complaints among Elderly Persons: An Epidemiologic Study of Three Communities." *Sleep* 18 (1995): 425–32.

CHAPTER 15: LOW GEAR—THE PROBLEMS OF SHIFT WORKERS

Carbone, John and Alex Kerin. "Financial Opportunities of Extended Hours Operations: Managing Costs, Risks and Liabilities. Circadian Technologies." Available from: http://www.circadian.com/publications/costs.html.

Olson, Leslie G. and Antonio Ambrogetti. "Working Harder—Working Dangerously? Fatigue and Performance in Hospitals." *Medical Journal of Australia* 168 (1998): 614–16.

Tenkanen L., T. Sjoblom, R. Kalimo, T. Alikoski, and M. Harma. Shift Work, Occupation and Coronary Heart Disease: Over Six Years of Follow-up in the Helsinki Heart Study. *Scandinavian Journal of Work and Environmental Health* 23, no. 4 (August 1997): 257–65.

Furlan, Raffaello, Franca Barbic, Simona Piazza, Mauro Tinelli, Paolo Seghizzi, and Alberto Malliani. "Modifications of Cardiac Autonomic Profile Associated with a Shift Schedule of Work." *Circulation* 102 (2000): 1912–16.

Weiss, Barbara. "Balancing Act: Taking on the Night Shift." *RN* 67 (August 1, 2004): 59.

1999 Sleep in Amerca Poll. National Sleep Foundation. Available from: http://www.sleepfoundation.org/publication/1999poll.cfm.

RESOURCES

www.sleepfoundation.org/disorder.cfm (National Sleep Foundation)
www.nhlbi.nih.gov (National Heart, Lung, and Blood Institute)
med.stanford.edu/school/psychiatry/narcolepsy (Narcolepsy information)
www.narcolepsynetwork.org (Narcolepsy information)
www.rls.org (Restless legs syndrome information)
www.stanford.edu/~dement/children.html (Children's sleep disorders)
www.sleepfoundation.org (Sleep disorders in women)
www.sleepapnea.org (American Sleep Apnea Association)
www.noah-health.org/en/sleep/concerns/elderly.html (Sleep disorders in the elderly)
www.kidshealth.org/kid/health_problems/teeth/snoring.html (Snoring in children)
www.dentalsleepmed.org (Oral appliance contact information)
www.virtualsleepclinic.com (Dr. Andrew Tucker Web site)
www.sleepresearchsociety.org
www.ESRS.org (EUROPEAN sleep society)
www.Neuronic.com/british.htm (British Sleep Society link)
www.css.to (Canadian Sleep Society)
www.british-sleep-society.org.uk
www.awakeinamerica.org
www.sleepaus.on.net (Australasian Sleep Association)

INDEX

Page numbers in *italics* refer to charts and illustrations

acid reflux, 172
actigraphy, 272–73
adenoids, 70, 75, 79, 121, 178, 217, 218
advanced sleep phase syndrome (ASPS), 247–49, 258
Afrin, 108
agomelatine (Valdoxan), *187*
airflow, 17, 63, 67, 76, *77,* 105, 106
    test for, 76–77
airways, 67, 68, 69, 70, 72, 74, 80, 84, 98, 105–6, 111, 115, 120, 133, 217, 232, 236, 240
alcohol, 11, 16, 37, 43, 52, 55, 62, 70, 93, 104, 125, 136, *141,* 149, 157, 158, 171, 174, 176, 177, 180, 204, 205, 236, 241, 243, 249, 251, 260, 275
alcoholism, 92, 202
Alertec, *see* modafinil
Allegra, 170

Allerest, 108
allergic rhinitis, 107–9, 178, 218
allergies, 4, 42, 67, 70, 74, 78, 79, 84, 98, 104, 106, 108, 109, 110, 115, 176
    of children, 208, 217–19
allergy pills, 107–8
alternative remedies, 149–50
Alzheimer's disease, 163, 176, 250, 251
Ambien (zolpidem), 184, *185, 187,* 200, 229
Ambrogetti, Antonio, 267, 269
American Academy of Sleep Medicine, 66, 204
Americans with Disabilities Act, 271
amnesia, sleep-related, 20
amphetamines, 128, 143, 275
Anafranil (clomipramine), *141,* 145
anemia, 157, 158, 163, 164

Antarctica, 268–69
antidepressants, 176, *185,* 190, 202, 230,
    237, 238, 250–51, 275
  for narcolepsy, 145–47
antihistamines, 55, 107, 109–10, 170, *185,*
    218, 251, 259
antiseizure drugs, 148, 157, 206
anxiety, 26, 49, 155, 156, 172, 177, 178,
    180, 202, 230, 234, 253
  in partners of snorers, 65
apnea index, 86–87
Army, U.S., 9, 115
arousal disorders, 195–99
arrhythmia, 119, 120
  sleep apnea and, 93, 100
arthritis, 139, 156, 176, 180, 237, 249
asthma, 11, 79, 98, 108, 176, 195
atomoxetine (Strattera), *141*
atonia, 2, 21–22, 31, 194, 200, 201–2
attention-deficit hyperactivity disorder
    (ADHD), 5, 95–96, 143, 156, 176,
    214–17, 219, 223
auditory hallucinations, 134

baby boomers:
  aging parents of, 241–42
  retirement by, 25, 189, 242–43
bariatric surgery, 2, 126
baths, 14, 41, 46, 159, 171, 200, 244
Bayer PM, *185*
bed partners, 31
  CPAP machines and, 103
  parasomnias and, 199, 204, 205–6
  PLMD and, 160
  sleep apnea and, 10, 84, 88, 102–3
  sleep medicine and observations by, 4
  snoring and, 3, 4, 27, 63, 64–65, 80
bedrooms, 41–42, 182, 221, 236, 241, 259
bedtime, 37, 38, 39, 40, 45, 158
bedtime rituals, 44, 45–46, 48, 198
  for children, 45, 221
Begin, Menachem, 33
behavioral sleep problems, 24, 37–38, 53
behavioral therapy, 123, 142, 149, 175, 192,
    200, 202, 229, 237, 238
  for insomnia, 182–83, 190–91
Benadryl, 109, 170, *185,* 218, 250
benzodiazepines, 159, 184, *185,* 188, 199,
    200, 202, 206, 254, 257
beta-blockers, 176, 251

biological clock, 28, 29, 40, 43, 60, 230
  at various ages, 22–23, 211, 243–46, *244,*
    245, 246, 258
blood flow, 44, 97–98, 158, 200
blood-oxygen levels, 86, 90
blood pressure, 22, 86, 92, 94, 139, 166,
    182, 194, 238
  high, 11, *63,* 82, 92, 93, 100, 143, 145
blood vessels, 69, 97, 107
body position therapy, 124–25
bones, facial, 66, 71, 91, 104, 112, 121
brain, 30, 87, 99, 138, 168
brain waves, 17, 20, 21
breast feeding, 107, 148, 233
Breathe Right Strips, 110–11
breathing:
  cessation of, *see* sleep apnea
  deep, 41
  in REM sleep, 21
breathing disorder index, 119
breathing disorders, 13, 16, 79
breathing rate, 76
bright light therapy, 230, 258–59, 276
bromocriptine (Parlodel), 254
bronchoconstriction, 98
bronchodilators, 250
Bruce, Lenny, 128–29
bruxism (teeth grinding), 112
bupropion, 176
Burdine, Calvin, 88–89

caffeine, 43, 44, 157, 158, 176, 178, 210,
    221, 230, 233, 236, 241, 251, 273, 275
calcium, 230
cancer, 55, 176
Cannon, Joe, 88–89
carbamazepine (Tegretol), 148, 159, 254
carbidopa, 159, 254
carbon dioxide, 17, 86, 87
cardiovascular disease, 4, 80, 92–93, 100,
    253
cardiovascular system, 11
cataplexy, 132, 133, 134, 137, 138, 140,
    142, 151, 201
  treatment for, *141,* 145, 146
Celexa (citalopram), 146
Center for Corrective Jaw Surgery, 102
cerebral cortex, 166
children, 22, 208–23
  ADHD in, 214–17, 219, 223

allergies of, 208, 217–19
amounts of sleep needed by, 209
bedtime rituals and routines for, 45, 221
bedtimes of, 209–12
decongestants and, 107
disoriented arousals in, 220
narcolepsy in, 16, 219
obesity in, 16, 208
parasomnias in, 219–21
rhythmic movement disorder in, 200, 220
RLS in, 158
sleep apnea in, 213–14, 218
sleep deprivation of, 16
sleep disordered breathing in, 213–14, 216
sleep terrors in, 196, 220–21
sleepwalking in, 197, 220
snoring by, 79, 208, 216, 221
weight of, 208, 213, 222
Children's Depression Inventory, 214
chocolate, 44, 222, 251
choking, 51, 97
cholesterol, high, 80, 100
chronic fatigue syndrome, 140, 180, 237
chronic obstructive pulmonary disease (COPD), 255
circadian rhythms, 28, 36–37, 40, 55, 127, 130, 243
eagles and, 58, 226
shift workers and, 55, 265–67, 270, 271, 276–77
sleep apnea and, 97–98
circadian sleep disorders:
behavioral, 266
endogenous, 266
temporal, 266–67
Circadian Technologies, 264–65
citalopram (Celexa), 146
Claritin, 170, 218
clomipramine (Anafranil), 141, 145
clonazepam (Klonopin), 159, 202, 206, 254, 257
Cloward, Tom V., 94
codeine, 148, 159, 254
coffee, 16, 37, 43, 47, 48, 136, 170, 176, 178, 249, 268
cognitive therapy, 48, 175, 183–84, 190–92, 200, 202, 229
colds, see allergic rhinitis

concentration, 10, 54, 269
confusional arousals, 196, 203, 220
congestive heart failure (CHF), 11, 84, 98, 255
Connor, James, 162–63
coronary artery disease, 11, 94, 99
corticosteroids, 250
cortisol, 143, 177, 270
costs:
of shift work, 265
of sleep apnea, 12
of sleep loss medically, 10–11
of sleep loss to employers, 10
of tired motorists, 14
of tired truckers, 14–15
CPAP (continuous positive air pressure) machine, 27, 56, 91, 93, 94, 95, 97, 99, 100, 102, 103, 116–24, 236, 240–41
CPAP mask (interface), 118, 119, 122
cromolyn sodium, 110
Cunningham, John, 52
Cylert (pemoline), 141, 145

Dalmane (flurazepam), 185, 187
darkness, 40, 41, 43
daylight, see sunlight
daylight savings time, 29, 225
day people, see larks
Day Reconstruction Model, 238
daytime, sleep issues connected to, 24–26, 48–49, 50
decongestants, 107, 250, 251
deep sleep, 23, 227–28
growth hormone and, 22, 246–47
delayed sleep phase syndrome (DSPS), 32, 247–49
delta waves, 21, 194
Dement, William, 33
dental appliances, 112–14, 116, 236
Dental Sleep Society, 114
deprenyl (selegiline; Eldepryl), 141, 145
depression, 5, 11, 26, 55, 65, 96, 129, 155, 230, 233, 235, 240
insomnia and, 55, 177, 178, 180, 185, 252
narcolepsy and, 135–36, 140
sleep apnea and, 96, 101, 102, 240–41
desipramine, 198, 202
Desosyn (methamphetamine), 141, 144
deviated septums, 75, 76, 77–78, 79, 106, 111–12, 120

dextroamphetamine (Dexedrine), *141,* 144
diabetes, 5, 11, 22, *63,* 65, 92, 107, 126, 139, 157, 158
    sleep apnea and, 95, 100, 101
diazepam, 159, 199, 206
diet, 13, 44, 127, 149, 181, 230, 257, 258, 268, 274
    poor, 24, 127
diuretics, 251, 257
DME (durable medical equipment) companies, 117, 122
dopamine, 145, 159, 253
Doppler sonography, 69, 158, 199–200
Doral (quazempam), *187*
dreams, dreaming, 19, 132, 142, 194, 201–2, 203–4
    muscle paralysis during, 2, 21–22, 31, 132
dream sleep, *see* REM sleep
drivers, 9, 13–15, 30, 151
dry mouth, 77, 83
dust mites, 98, 110
dysesthesias, 155

eagles, 58, 225, 226, 247
ear, nose, and throat specialists (ENTs), 2, 81, 98, 109, 111, 113, 115, 237
earplugs, 41, 65
eating disorders, 136
echocardiograms, 100, 144
Edison, Thomas, 43, 60, 142
Edronex (reboxetine), *141,* 147
EDS (excessive daytime sleepiness), *51,* 52–56, 60, *63,* 70, 80, 89, 96, 120, 133, 136, 139, 140, *141,* 144, 163–64, 178, 201, 225, 232, 238, 242, 249
EDT, 162
Effexor (venlafaxine), *141,* 146
Ehrlich, Paul, 218
Elavil (imipramine), *141,* 145, *185*
Eldepryl (selegiline; deprenyl), *141,* 145
elderly, 240–61
    insomnia in, 177, 182
    sunlight and, 43
electrocardiograms (ECGs), 100, 269
electrocortical arousals, 120
electroencephalograms (EEGs), 19, 80, 130, 132, 183
electromyography, 158
Endep, *185*

endothelial cells, 69
Enovil, *185*
ENS (excessive nighttime sleepiness), for owls, 60
ephedrine, 108, 150
epilepsy, 137
epinephrine, 133
Epworth Sleepiness Scale, 11, *51, 52,* 55–56
erectile tissue, 22, 102–3, 194
esophageal reflux, *54*
estazolam (ProSom), *185, 187*
estrogen, 226, 234
eszopiclone (Lunesta), *187,* 189
evolution, circadian rhythms and, 37
ExcedrinPM, *185*
exercise, 36, 43, 56, 127, 151, 159, 181, 233, 240, 257, 273, 276
    appropriate times for, 44, 174, 258
    by children, 213
    lack of, 5, 11, 16, 24, 65, 125
    relaxation, 41, 44, 182, 198
eye movements, 20, 21–22, 194
eyes, 28, 40, 265
eye shades, 41

face, bones of, 66, 71, 91, 104, 112, 121
facial structure, 70, *71*
fat, 44
Federal Motor Carrier Safety Administration (FMCSA), 14
fetal growth reduction, 232
fiberscope, 111
fibromyalgia, 176
fight-or-flight response, 85, 133, 166, 167
fixed blockages, 110–12
fluoxetine (Prozac), *141,* 146, 176, 251
fluphenazine, 198
flurazepam (Dalmane), *185, 187*
folate, 158, 237
food, fast, 65, 101, 125, 221
Food and Drug Administration (FDA), 112, 113, 117, 147, 150, 188
football players:
    nasal dilators worn by, 76
    sleep apnea levels of, 2, 89–90, 91
Freud, Sigmund, 19, 31
frontalis muscle tension, 168
Furlan, Raffaello, 270

GABA (gamma-aminobutyric acid), 188
gabapentin, 159
gaboxadol, *187*
gamma-hydroxybutyrate (GHB), 147
Gangwisch, James, 13
gastric bypass, 126
gastroesophageal reflux disorder (GERD),
    98–99
gastroplasty, 126
genetics:
    in insomnia, 178
    narcolepsy and, 139
    sleep and, 39
    sleep schedules and, 57
    of snoring, 74, 81
ghrelin, 13
glucose, 168, 268
Gozal, David, 217
growth spurt, 22
guided imagery, 123

Halcion (triazolam), *185, 187*
Hall, Jim, 14–15
hallucinations, 134
haloperidol, 157
headaches, *51,* 83, 99, 100, 101, 195
hearing, snoring and, 65, 68
heart, 11, 97, 99, 146, 255–57
heart attacks, 69, 84, 98, 100, 260
heart disease, 5, 12, 22, *63,* 88, 92,
    101, 104, 107, 120, 176, 184, 236, 249
    snoring and, 65
    valvular, 144
heart failure, 11, 91, 180
heart rate, 17, 22, 86, 139, 182, 194
Heavy Snorer's Disease, 80–81
Heimlich maneuver, 83, 84, 87
Helsinki Heart Study, 268
HEPA (high-efficiency purification
    apparatus) filters, 110
herbal remedies, *186,* 251
herbal tea, 46, 52
Heyman, Charles, 26
Heymsfield, Steven, 13
Hirshkowitz, Max, 102–3
histamines, 109, 110, 133, 170
HLA (human leukocyte antigen), 139,
    140
hormone replacement therapy,
    234

hormones, 5, 22, 91, 103, 225, 226, 228, 236
hospital nurseries, 16, 211
hot flashes, 234
hours-of-service (HOS) regulations, 14
human growth hormone (HGH), 22, 143,
    246–47
hyperarousal, 172
hypersomnia, 52, 228
hypertension, 5, 11, *63,* 80, 92, 120, 126,
    176, 232, 236, 243
    sleep apnea and, 93, 94
    snoring and, 65, 80
hyperthyroidism, 176, 178
hypertonic saline solutions, 108, 109
hypnagogic hallucinations, 133–34, 145,
    201
hypnic jerks, 20
hypnosis, 199
hypnotics, *see* sleeping pills
hypocretin, 139, 148, 150, 167
hypoglycemia, 129
hypopharynx, 66, *66,* 78, *78*
hypopnea, *63, 63*
hypothalamus, 28, 138, 139, 234
hypothyroidism, 55, 252

idiopathic pulmonary fibrosis (IPF),
    146
illness, sleeping problems and, 37, 38,
    54–55, 249–50
imagery training, 183
imipramine (Elavil; Janimine; Tofranil),
    141, 145, 185
immune system, 19, 109
immunotherapy desensitization, 110
impotence, *51,* 83
Indiplon, *187*
infants, 16, 22, 211
insomnia, 3, 16, 23, 42–43, 136, 156, 162,
    165–92, 222, 238, 272
    acute, 175, 181
    age and, 172, 252, 254, 256, 258
    anxiety and, 49, 174
    behavioral changes and, 169, 170
    causes of, 37–38, 46–47, 168–69, 170,
        172–74, 176–78
    chronic, 47, 176, 179, 188, 192, 230
    days as key to, 47–48
    depression and, 55, 177, 178, 180, *185,*
        252

insomnia (*continued*)
EDS vs., 52
idiopathic, 179
intermittent (short-term), 175
menopause and, 235
in partners of snorers, 65
PMS and, 228
primary, 165–66, 178–79
psychophysiologic, 179
retirement and, 25, 47, 189–91
secondary, 165–66, 176–78, 184
self-medication for, 171, 174, 180–81
sleep maintenance, 155, 172
sleep onset, 155, 172
three P's model of, 173, 235
treatment for, 169, 170, 175, 176, 178, 179–84, *185–87*, 188–89
types of, 175–76
waking time management and, 5
insulin, 95, 268-69
insurance, 3–4, 112, 115, 143
intubation, 84, 99
iron, 157, 158, 162–63, 164, 237
isotonic saline solutions, 108

Janimine (imipramine), *141*, 145, *185*
Japan, 90
jaw:
lower, 71–72, 79, 121
surgery on, 124
jet lag, 175, 266–67, 268
Johns, Murray, *51*

Kahneman, Daniel, 238
KGB, 33, 34
kidney failure, 157, 180
kidney problems, 158
Kindred, Audrey, 152
Klonopin (clonazepam), 159, 202, 206, 254, 257

Lacasse, Yves, 96
larks, 57–58, *59*, 60, 226, 247, 265–66
L-dopa (levodopa), 159, 219, 253, 254
leg movement disorders, 16, 160, 195, *238*, 239, 272
legs, muscle activity in, 17
leptin, 13
level 1, *66, 78*, 79, 104, 105–6, 107–12, 116–23

level 2, *66, 78*, 79, 104, 112–15, 116–23
level 3, *66, 78*, 79, 112–14, 116–23, 124
levodopa (L-dopa), 159, 219, 253, 254
Levy, Allan M., 90
light, 28, 41, 181, 236, 241, 265
light boxes, 230, 259
limb movement disorders, *see* leg movement disorders
Lisanby, Sarah, 26
locking jaw, 72
lorazepam, 199
Louis Harris and Associates, Inc., 9–10
lower jaw, 70, 104, 106, 112–13
Lunesta (eszopiclone), *187*, 189
lung disease, 84, 88, 100, 104, 120, 146, 176, 184, 249
lungs, 11, 98, 99, 255–57

Maas, James B., 43
McDonnell, Maggie, 14
McGlasson, Robert, 88–89
macroglossia, 72
Maggie's Law, 14
magnesium, 158
magnetic resonance imagery (MRI), 26
mandible, 66, 112
retroplaced, 124
mandibular advancing devices, 112–13, 124
massages, 159, 200, 233
maxilla, 66, 112
Medicare, 119
medications, 70, 104, 123, 142, 192, 198, 235, 238, 275, 277
EDS and, 54, 55
in elderly, 250–51, 259–60
insomnia and, 175, 176, 181, 184, *185–87*, 188–89
for narcolepsy, 137
RLS and, 157, 159
meditation, 198
MEDWATCH, 150
melatonin, 28, 143, *186*, 188, 259, 276
memory, 23, 269
men:
insomnia in, 171, 179, 225
PLMD in, 160
REM sleep disorders in, 202
RLS in, 156, 232
sleep apnea in, 82, 84, 92, 226

menopause, 180, 226, 234–37
menstrual cycle, 226–30, 234
metabolism, 4, 139, 254, 259
methamphetamine (Desosyn), *141,* 144
methylphenidate (Ritalin), 95, *141,* 143, 144, 214–16
metoclopramide, 157
microsleeps, 135, 249
military, extended waking in, 26
milk, 44, 171, 174
Miltown, 184
Mirapex (pramipexole), 159, 164, 253, 254
modafinil (Provigil; Alertec), 133, *141,* 142–44, 275
monoamine oxidase B, 145
monoamine oxidase inhibitors, 145–46
Morin, Charles, 174
motor movements, abnormal, *54*
motor restlessness, 156
mouth breathing, 77–78
mucous membranes, 69, 78
multiple sclerosis, 15, 55, 132, 139, 202
multiple sleep latency test (MSLT), 56–57, 140, 142, 272
muscle activity, 17, 21, 139
muscle repair, 91
muscles, voluntary, 124
muscle tone, 132, 133
Myers, Janet, 103
myocardial disease, 12, 99

naps, 38, 43, *51,* 83, 136, 149, 151, 174–75, 176, 233, 249, 274
    forced, *141,* 142
narcolepsy, 15, 25, 43, 54, 128–52, 160, 201, 272
    age and, 15, 129–30, 137–38
    in animals, 131, 138, 139, 148–49
    in children, 16, 219
    diagnosis of, 56, 136, 139–40
    management of, 5, 151–52
    quality of life and, 137–38
    symptoms of, 130–31, 133–36, 138
    treatment for, 140, *141,* 142–50
    work and, 136–37, 140, 151
Narcolepsy Network, 152
nares, 76
NasalCrom, 110
nasal sprays, 107–8

nasal valve dilators, 76, 110–11
nasopharynx, 66, *66,* 75–76, 78, *78,* 79, 104, 107, 115, 218
National Heart, Lung and Blood Institute (NHLBI), 65–66, 255
National Institute on Aging, 141
National Sleep Foundation (NSF), 9–10, 25, 66, 91, 210, 221, 225, 230, 237, 274
"natural" remedies, 149–50
neck, 70, 74, 79, 82, 91, 101, 104, 106
Neo-Synephrine, 108
nerve conduction studies, 158
nervous system, 11, 22, 69, 166, 169, 179
    autonomic, 166–67, 168, 195
    enteric, 166
    sympathetic, 85, 86, 133
neural pathways, 13, 19
neurochemical pathways, 5, 39, 169
neurons, 22, 26
neuropathology, 202
neuropathways, 147, 169
neuropathy, peripheral, 157, 158
neuroproteins, 138
neurotonin, 234
neurotransmitters, 5, 132, 139, 150, 159, 166, 169, 188, 234
New York Methodist Hospital, 3, 126, 173
    sleep center at, 3, 10–11, 16–17, 79
    Web site sleep test of, 7–8, 17
NFL, 89–90
nicotine, 43, 176, 178, 181, 251, 260, 273
nightmares, 31, 200–201, 220
    waking, 136
night people, *see* owls
night shift work, *see* shift work
night terrors, *see* sleep terrors
nighttime sleep-related eating disorder, 237–38
nocturnal leg cramps, 199–200
noise, 41, 181, 241
non-REM sleep, 20–21, 24, 39, 46, 131–32, *185,* 193, 194, 206, 212, 246
nonsteroidal anti-inflammatories (NSAIDs), 250
norepinephrine, 132–33, 146, 166, 167, 168, 180, 188, 234
nose, 66, 70, 75, 105, 106–7, 111, 120
nurses, shift work and, 271
Nytol, *185*

obesity, 11, 13, *63,* 74, 125–26, 178
    childhood, 16
    snoring and, 70, 80
    see also weight
obsessing, 40–41, 169
obstructive sleep apnea (OSA), *see* sleep
    apnea
Olson, Leslie, 267, 269
opiates, 148, 254
opioids, 159
optic nerves, 28, 41
orexins, 133, 138, 139, 140, 149
oropharnyx, 66, *66,* 74, 78, *78*
oropharynx surgery, 114–16
orthodontists, 2, 113, 114
otolaryngologists, *see* ear, nose, and throat
    specialists
owls, 57–58, *59,* 60, 226, 247, 263, 265–66,
    271
oxazempam (Serax), *187*
oxycodone (Roxicodone), 159, 254
oxygen, 17, 69, 86, 87, 88, 91, 95, 99, 120,
    256–67
oxymetazoline, 107–8

palate, 70, 74, 79, 104, 106, 112, 114
paradoxical intention, 192
parasomnias, 16, 26, 88, 193–207, 252
    arousal disorders, 195–99
    REM sleep, 195, 200–202
    sexual aggression in sleep, 203, 205–6
    sleep-wake transition disorders, 195,
        199–200
    violence in sleep, 203–5, 206
parasthesias, 155
Parents Against Tired Truckers, 14
Parkinson's disease, 55, 70, 129, 137, 157,
    159, 163, 164, 176, 202, 219, 250,
    252–53
Parlodel (bromocriptine), 254
Paxil (paroxetine), *141*
Pediatric Quality of Life Inventory, 214
pemoline (Cylert), *141, 145*
PEP (Participate, Educate, and Propagate
    information), *141*
pergolide mesylate (Permax), 159, 254
periodic limb movement disorder
    (PLMD), 155, 156, 159, 160–63, 164,
    219, 237, 242, 253–54
Periodic Limb Movement Index, 161

peripheral vision, 30
Permax (pergolide mesylate), 159, 254
perphenazine, 198
personality changes, *51, 83*
pharyngeal mucosa, 69
pharynx, 67, 69, 70, 86, 114
phenobarbitol, 184
phenothiazine, 157
phenylephrine, 108
phenytoin, 157
Pickwickian syndrome, 91
Pickwick Postdoctoral Sleep Research
    Fellowships, 91
pineal gland, 28, 276
polyps, nasal, 70, 77, 79, 104, 106, 111–12,
    120
polysomnogram (PSG), 16, 140, 158, 196
positron-emission tomography (PET) scan,
    29–30, 168
posterior pharyngeal wall, 73
postnasal drip, 67
post-traumatic stress disorder, 202
power naps, 43
pramipexole (Mirapex), 159, 164, 253, 254
pregnancy, 107, 148, 157, 211, 226,
    230–33, 237, 238
premenstrual dysphoric disorder (PMDD),
    228–29
premenstrual syndrome (PMS), 225,
    228–29
prochlorperazine, 157
progesterone, 226, 228, 231, 234, 236
propoxyphene, 159
ProSom (estazolam), *185, 187*
protriptyline (Vivactil), *141,* 145
Provigil, *see* modafinil
Prozac (fluoxetine), *141,* 146, 176, 251
pseudoephedrine, 108, 251
psychiatric conditions, 5, 180, 251–52
psychological problems:
    dreams and, 19
    narcolepsy falsely associated with,
        129
    sleep, 24
psychotherapy, 194, 201, 235, 237
pulmonary edema, 99

Q-T interval change, 100, 226
quazempam (Doral), *187*
quinine, 200

ramelteon, *187*
rapid eye movement (REM), 17
rapid eye movement (REM) sleep, *see* REM sleep
reading, 41, 46, 174, 259
reboxetine (Edronax), *141,* 147
recklessness, 14, 30
red blood cells, 86
refocusing, 48–49
relaxation exercises, 41, 44
REM (rapid eye movement) sleep, 2, 19, 21–22, 24, 30–31, 39, 46, 56, 72, 76, 77, 80, 124, 131, 142, 152, 177, *185,* 193, 194, 195, 225, 234, 244–46, 263, 275
    atonia during, 2, 21–22, 31, 194, 200, 201
    of infants and children, 22, 212, 220, 244
    in narcolepsy, 129, 130, 132, 134, 142, 145
REM rebound, 201
REM sleep behavior disorder, 160, 198, 201–2, 206, 257
REM sleep parasomnias, 195, 200–202
ResMed Inc., 89
restless legs syndrome (RLS), 15, 54, 153–64, *161,* 178, 199, 232, 233, 237, 242
    causes of, 157
    in children, 16, 158
    diagnosing, 154, 155–56, 157–58
    in elderly, 252, 253–55
    family history in, 163–64
    idiopathic, 158
    treatment for, 158–59
Restless Legs Syndrome Foundation, 154, 156, 163, 255
Restoril (temazepam), *185, 187,* 206
retirement, insomnia during, 25, 47, 189–91
Rhone-Poulenc Rorer, 171
rhythmic movement disorder, 100, 220
Ritalin (methylphenidate), 95, *141,* 143, 144, 214–16
ropinirole hydrochloride, 159
Roxicodone (oxycodone), 159, 254

saline solution, 107, 108–9, 110
Saltaire, 109
Scheffler, William, 270–71

schizophrenia, 134, 180
sclerosis, 115
sedatives, 125, 177, 243
seizures, 195, 206
selective noradrenaline reuptake inhibitors, 147
selective serotonin reuptake inhibitors (SSRIs), 146–47, 250
selegiline (deprenyl, Eldepryl), *141,* 145
self-medication, 140, 171, 174, 180–81, 243
Serax (oxazempam), *187*
serotonin, 133, 146, 170, 234
serotonin reuptake inhibitors (SSRIs), *185,* 234
sertraline (Zoloft), *141*
sex, 102–3, 131
sexual aggression, in sleep, 203, 205–6
shift work, 9, 12, 28, 57–58, *141,* 231, 248, 262–77
    insomnia and, 177, 178
    variable, 271, 277
shift work sleep disorder, 271
Siegel, Jerome M., 170
siestas, 28, 36–37, 131
Silva, Jorge Alberto Costa E., 173–74
Simemet (carbidopa-levodopa), 254
Singulair, 218
sinuses, 78, 105–6
sinusitis, 79, 120–21
sleep:
    amounts of, 39, 151
    anchor, 274
    continuous, 39, 80
    daily need of, 39–40
    daytime issues and, 24–26
    disrupted, 39, 238
    needs at various ages, 22–23
    patterns of, 158
    preparation for, 36, 37–38, 44–46
    as restorative, 22, 46, 80, 91, 227–28
    split, 274
    unusual schedules vs., 31–32
sleep aids, over-the-counter, 171, *185,* 259
sleep apnea, 2, 54, 56–57, 63, *63,* 67, 68, 80, 82–104, *87,* 110, 133, 159, 164, 165, 178, 195, 263, 272
    age and, 82, 92, 240–41, 242, 243, 252–53, 256
    in children, 213–14
    as cofactor in diseases, 11, 92–96

sleep apnea (*continued*)
  costs of, 12, 101
  detection and prevalence of, 4, 10–11,
    54, 82–83, 96, 180
  heart conditions and, 99–100
  obstructive, *see* obstructive sleep apnea
  in pregnant women, 232
  sexual problems from, 102–3
  treatment for, 105–27
  weight and, 13, 56, 82, 84, 90, 91, 93,
    95–96, 104, 125–27, 240
sleep attacks, 130
sleep bingeing, 16
sleep centers, 101, 122, 136, 140, 179–80
  development of, 2
  at Methodist Hospital, 3, 10–11, 16–17,
    79
sleep cycles, length of, 22
sleep deficit, 9, 29, 53, 201, 225, 242, 269
  in women, 225, 226
sleep deprivation, 56, 198, 205, 243, 267
  EDS and, 53–54
  effects on brain of, 29–30
  in partners of snorers, 65
  as torture, 33, 34
sleep diaries, 38, 179, 222, 229, 261, 272,
    279, *280–87*
sleep-disordered breathing, 63, *63,* 238
  in children, 213–14
  in menopause, 235–36
sleep disorders:
  EDS and, 54
  genetic factors in, 4
  insomnia caused by, 178
  knowledge of, 2
  prevalence of, 9–11
  societal costs of, 9–11
  subjective suspicions of, 52
  in those who sleep alone, 4, 23, 31
  see also specific disorders
sleep homeostasis, 29
sleep hygiene, 32, 38–39, 46–48, 60, 127,
    137, *141,* 142, 164, 176, 181, 182, 183,
    192, 201, 230, 235, 236, 249, 254, 257,
    272, 273
sleepiness:
  excessive daytime, *see* EDS (excessive
    daytime sleepiness)
  normal vs. abnormal,
    53–54

sleeping pills (hypnotics), *141,* 175, 177,
    184, 190, 200, 260, 275
  non-prescription, *185*
sleep insufficiency, EDS and, 53–54
sleep maintenance insomnia, 155
sleep medicine, as new and evolving
    specialty, 1–5, 11, 16, 27–28, 31
sleep onset insomnia, 155
sleep paralysis, 134–35, 136, 145, 201
sleep positions, 72, 80, 104, 233, 263
sleep rebound, 201
sleep-related abnormal swallowing
    syndrome, 195
sleep-related amnesia, 20
sleep restriction, 183, 230
Sleep Societies Worldwide, 66
sleep stages, 20–22, 194
  of adults, *20, 244, 245*
  of children, *21, 244*
  of elderly, *246*
  non-REM, *see* non-REM sleep
  REM sleep, *see* rapid eye movement
    sleep
  stage 1, 20, 194
  stage 2, 20, 194, 267
  stage 3, 21, 194
  stage 4, 21, 194
sleep starts, 199
sleep state misperception disorder, 172,
    179
sleep studies, 115, 158
sleep talking, 16, 199, 220
Sleep Tech Consulting Group, 89
sleep terrors, 196–97, 198, 200, 220–21
sleep-wake arousal systems, 139
sleep-wake behavior, 138
sleep-wake cycle, 168, 188, 222, 265
  naps as disrupting to, 43
sleep-wake disorder, 90
sleep-wake schedules, irregular, 176
sleep-wake transition disorders, 195,
    199–200
sleepwalking, 16, 26, 195, 197–98, 203, 237
  in children, 197, 220
smoking, 5, 11, 38, 43, 62, 70, 92, 93, 100,
    101, 136, 157, 158, 176, 260, 268
snoring, 3, 17, *51,* 61–82, 110, 164, 236,
    238, 242, 263
  bed partners and, 3, 4, 27, 63, 64–65, 80
  by children, 79, 208, 216, 221

complicated, 63
damage caused by, 2, 4, 62–63, 64–66, 68–70, 80
indicators for, 66–68, 70–71
in pregnant women, 232
self-examination for, 61–62
simple, 63, 63
treatment for, 63–65, 105–27
social interaction, 23, 178
"social sleeping," 37, 42
sodium oxybate (Xyrem), 141, 147–48
soft palate, 66, 73, 104, 112, 263
soft tissue, 66, 104
Sominex, 185
somnabulism, see sleepwalking
Sonata (zaleplon), 185, 187
Sopranos, The, 89, 101
Spielman, Arthur J., 173, 183
spouses, see bed partners
Stern, Yaakov, 26
stimulants, 142–45
Strattera (atomoxetine), 141
stress, 10, 24, 25, 26, 47, 95, 133, 156, 175, 181, 182, 198, 201, 205, 268
stressors, 167, 172, 176–78, 179, 180, 228
stroke, 22, 69, 70, 94, 236, 253, 260
substance abuse, 5, 55, 136–37, 177, 178
sudden infant death syndrome (SIDS), 213
sumo wrestlers, 90
sunlight, 40, 43, 258
suprachiasmatic nucleus (SCN), 28, 211, 243, 259, 265
Suzuki, Naohito, 90

tea, 43
    herbal, 46, 52
teenagers, 16, 29, 266
    growth spurt of, 22
Tegretol (carbamazepine), 148, 159, 254
television, 33, 34, 40, 41, 44, 48, 182, 221–22, 259
temazepam (Restoril), 185, 187, 206
temperature:
    of bedroom, 42, 181, 236, 241
    body, 36–37, 168, 270
testosterone, 103, 227
tetradecyl sulfate, 115
theophylline, 176
thioridazine, 198
throat, 66, 73

thyroid, 180
TMJ (temporomandibular joint) problems, 72, 112, 114
tobacco, see smoking
Tofranil (imipramine), 141, 145, 185
tongue, 66, 67, 70, 72, 79, 80, 84, 87, 104, 106, 112–13, 115, 121, 124
tongue-retaining devices, 112–13
tonsillectomies, 218
tonsils, 66, 70, 75, 79, 106, 178, 208, 217
    "kissing," 104, 121
torture, sleep deprivation as, 33, 34
toxic environment, 5
tracheostomy, 84
tracheotomy, 84, 116
traffic accidents, 9, 13–15, 30, 52, 56, 89, 274–75
tranquilizers, 251
transcranial magnetic stimulation (TMS), 26
triacylglycerol (TAG), 269
triazolam (Halcion), 185, 187
truckers, 14–15, 58
tumors, 30, 106, 116, 120, 121, 123
24/7 business environment, 12, 40, 58, 263
tyramine, 145

Unisom, 185
United States Defense Advanced Research Projects Agency (DARPA), 26
upper airway resistance syndrome, 80
urination, 51, 96–97, 109, 231, 250
uvula, 66, 67, 73, 79, 84, 87, 106, 112, 114
uvulopalatopharyngoplasty (UPPP), 114–15

Valdoxan (agomelatine), 187
valium, 55
vasoactive rhinitis, 120
venlafaxine (Effexor), 141, 146
Vicks Sinex, 108
viloxazine, 145
violence, in sleep, 203–5, 206
Vivactil (protriptyline), 141, 145
vocal cords, 98, 111, 123

wake times, 38, 40, 41
Walter Reed Army Institute of Research, 26
weekends, sleeping patterns and, 37, 42

weight, 44, 67, 178, 225, 236
  of children, 208, 213, 222
  insomnia and, 167, 178
  sleep apnea and, 13, 56, 82, 84, 90, 91,
    93, 95–96, 104, 125–27, 240
Weiss, Barbara, 271
"white noise" machines, 41
Winstead, Liz, 138
women, 224–39
  as eagles, 225, 226
  EDS in, 225, 232
  insomnia in, 171–72, 179, 224–25, 228,
    229–30, 235
  PLMD in, 160
  REM sleep disorders in, 202
  RLS in, 156, 232
  sleep apnea in, 82, 92, 225, 226, 236, 239
  sleep deficit in, 225, 226

  see also menopause; menstrual cycle;
    pregnancy
work:
  day vs. night people and types of, 57
  EDS as hindrance to, 52–53, 56
  sleepiness at, 25, 56–57
worry, 49, 169, 178, 230
wrestlers, 168–69

Xyrem (sodium oxybate), *141,* 147–48

yoga, 44, 198

zaleplon (Sonata), *185, 187*
Zhu, Jin Liang, 231
Zoloft (sertraline), *141*
zolpidem (Ambien), 184, *185, 187,* 200
zopiclone, 189